THE ANXIETY CURE: 2-IN-1 BUNDLE

Social Anxiety Cure + Adult ADHD & ADD Solution - The #1 Complete Box Set to Restore Attention, Control Stress, and Overcome Shyness

The Social Anxiety Cure: Defeat Shyness & Anxiety Forever

Discover How to Reduce Stress and Prevent Depression in Just 7 Days, Even if You're Extremely Shy and Introverted

By Frank Steven

Table of Contents

Introduction 6
Chapter 1: Understanding Anxiety and Social Anxiety 8
    What Is Anxiety? 9
    How Fear Develops into Anxiety 11
    Fight or Flight of Anxiety 13
    Panic Attacks 15
    Social Anxiety and the Mind 16
    Myths About Social Anxiety 18
    When Social Anxiety Gets Serious 21
    What Is a Phobia? 22
Chapter 2: Managing Social Anxiety 26
    Rewiring the Thinking Patterns 26
    Boosting Self-Confidence 30
    Managing Self-Consciousness 33
Chapter 3: Social Anxiety in Daily Life 38
    Keeping the Mind Calm 40
    Managing Anxious Thoughts 44
    Managing the Panic Mind 47
    Overcoming Panic Attacks 49
    Managing Stress Levels 51
    Stress Inoculation Training – A Treatment for Social Anxiety 53
Chapter 4: Understanding Depression 56
    What Is Depression? 58
    Depression in the Mind 62
    Suicide – Myths of Suicide 65
    What Happens When Depression Gets Serious? 70
Chapter 5: Managing Depression 73
    Boost Your Self-Esteem 73
    The Healthy Brain (SEEDS) 76
    Socialization 77
    Education 80

Exercise..81
Diet 82
Sleep..83
Use of Self-Love and Self-Compassion 85
Practice Mindfulness – Be in the Moment 87
Chapter 6: Wrapping It Up – Strategies and Resources 91
Check Your Progression on Overcoming Social Anxiety
or Depression 91
Talk to Someone 95
Get Your Family and Friends On Board! 100
Organizations and Resources... 103
Conclusion..105

Introduction

Congratulations on Purchasing *The Social Anxiety Cure: Defeat Shyness & Anxiety Forever*—and thank you for doing so!

Depression and anxiety are common mental health concerns that affect millions of people of all ages, genders, and races. Each diagnosis is unique to the person, and there are many treatment options and combinations of treatments that can make a difference. Depression can be treated, and someone who is depressed can find a way out of it.

There are many misconceptions when it comes to understanding the nuances of depression, phobias, and anxiety disorders. These misconceptions often paint the illness in a negative light. The truth is that everyone has fears. Everyone feels stressed. Everyone has moments in which the demands of life weigh heavily on their shoulders. Depression has many causes, and no person with this diagnosis will have the same symptoms or reactions.

This guide is meant to be a helpful and informative book that explains these complicated diagnoses in simple terms. While a guide like this should not replace the advice of a trained medical or mental health professional, helping people understand what depression is and how it can be managed provides hope to those who struggle daily to overcome this condition.

The following chapters will provide an insight into depression and social anxiety—two of the most common mental health diagnoses—and will provide suggestions and tips on how to manage depression and social anxiety. Other chapters will discuss techniques that supplement a formal treatment plan and focus on achieving a healthy mind and body as well as how to best utilize family and friends to work towards the lifting of depression.

There is a portion of the book that talks about the seriousness of depression. It covers the consequences to health because of the depressed mind, and it talks about suicide and the myths that obstruct better understanding of this very real consequence of depression. Addictions and self-harm also manifest when depression is undiagnosed and untreated.

There are plenty of books on this subject on the market—thanks again for choosing this one! Every effort was made to ensure it is full of as much useful information as possible. Please enjoy!

Chapter 1: Understanding Anxiety and Social Anxiety

The mind is a marvelous part of the human experience. It controls life functions, and it stores memories—it allows us to learn, to speak, to see, to experience life. It processes emotions, allows us to reason, and carries recollections of our triumphs and our tragedies. Its capabilities are limitless.

It is also fragile. It can be influenced by trauma, by a chemical imbalance, or by an illness. Its instincts are designed to protect the human being from danger or threats—but sometimes, that response overwhelms. Sometimes, the apprehension a person has prevents them from taking an active role in life. Sometimes, things that used to matter don't matter anymore. Sometimes, friends and family members are shut out—and being alone becomes the only choice.

Anxiety and depression are two of the most prevalent mental health diagnoses. That means that people who have these concerns don't have to feel like they are alone. Others have struggled with similar issues; others have been overwhelmed by anxiety; others have found ways to manage the symptoms as well as the disorder.

An important consideration is that anxiety disorders are not the same for everyone. Each person is triggered by something different—depending on their own life experiences and self-consciousness.

What Is Anxiety?

Expectant parents feel anxious as they anticipate the birth of their child. A spouse is anxious to hear the update from a surgeon about whether the surgery to remove a cancerous tumor went well. A high school student is anxious about stepping onto the stage to perform in the school's talent show. Passengers on an airplane feel a little anxious when turbulence is encountered.

Through the course of a day, a week, a month, a year, or even a lifetime—there will be many situations and circumstances that make a person anxious. Many of these are short-lived and cause no harm—rather, these worrisome moments assist the person in getting over fears as well as gaining confidence and experience to make it easier the next time around.

Anxiety is defined as a feeling of apprehension and fear. From a medical standpoint, these feelings of apprehension and fear are physically displayed by symptoms such as palpitations, sweating, and feelings of stress. Anxiety is a natural reaction—but if it becomes excessive, it can lead to more profound mental health issues and even impede someone from completing everyday tasks and responsibilities.
This serious reaction to anxiety is considered an anxiety disorder. This mental health concern afflicts an estimated 40 million adults in the United States. That is about 18 percent of the population. Eight percent of children and teens also suffer from an anxiety disorder of some type.

Anxiety disorders include: Generalized Anxiety Disorder which is excessive, constant worrying about the daily routine; Social Anxiety Disorder which is avoidance of social interactions in fear of being negatively judged or humiliated; Panic Disorder which is a physiological reaction brought on by feelings of terror; and phobias, which are an irrational fear of an object, place, or situation.

While the types of disorders vary, there are many common symptoms. In general, a person suffering from an anxiety disorder will have an unshakable and extreme fear or worry when this level of reaction is not necessary, such as when there is no threat or danger of physical harm.

Other commonplace emotional symptoms include restlessness, irritability, heightened awareness of the possibility of danger, tenseness, and a feeling of dread. On the physical side, a person will experience an increased heart rate, sweaty skin, headaches, shortness of breath, and gastrointestinal problems.

Anxiety disorders often mimic medical disorders, such as hyperthyroidism or heart conditions. Someone who is experiencing a panic attack and is undiagnosed with an anxiety disorder may think he or she is having a heart attack because of the similarities. Experts suggest that the first professional visit should be to a medical practitioner who can rule out medical reasons for the symptoms, followed by a referral to a mental health professional for an evaluation and plan of treatment.

Because anxiety disorders have unique characteristics, the treatment plans for these conditions is individualized. Routine treatments include psychotherapy, medications, and other techniques such as learning to reduce stress and foster relaxation.

How Fear Develops into Anxiety

Doctors cite two main sources for anxiety disorders – family genetics and life experiences. Evidence suggests that anxiety disorders tend to manifest generation to generation. If a family member, such as a parent, has an anxiety disorder, the risk of their offspring developing one greatly increases.

These psychological conditions can also come about from a traumatic experience, such as the death of a loved one, a long-lasting illness, an abusive relationship or exposure to violence of any kind.

But an anxiety disorder does not materialize overnight. It is a process that moves through stages and often spans years of experiences that contribute to the irrational fear. It is like a snowball that gathers both mass and force as it travels. A single incident is not likely to result in an anxiety disorder, but repeated exposure to similar incidents put a person at risk.

While family history tends to play a role, most research also suggests secondary sources as contributing to the development of anxiety disorders. These can include brain chemistry, life events and the personality of the afflicted person.

There could also be a medical reason for the events that build the anxiety levels a person will experience. Some of the medical reasons impacting anxiety include asthma, diabetes, drug abuse, heart disease, hormones, seizures, and thyroid conditions, to name a few. The first step in seeking an answer to the symptoms occurring is to seek the advice of a medical professional who can rule out other causes for the elevated fears and apprehensions.

Anxiety can also build up over time as a result of external factors. Some of the most common environmental causes include stress at work and school, marriage or relationship challenges, money troubles, substance abuse and a lack of oxygen.

The fear or worry experienced by a person could develop into an anxiety disorder over time. As the body releases hormones and prepares to confront the fear, it slows down some body functions in order to provide support to physical needs in fending off the threat.

Consider Post Traumatic Stress Disorder as an example of how prolonged exposure to fear can develop into a serious mental health issue. In war, soldiers witness extreme acts of violence, and they are constantly on high-alert. The adrenaline and other hormones which are designed to maximize responses in dangerous situations are at a continual high level.

The impacts of this on the physical body is that it weakens the body's natural defenses to ward off infection and hinders the immune system. Stomach and intestinal problems can wreak havoc on the physical wellbeing, as well as age the body more quickly.

Long-term exposure to fear also impairs the brain's ability to store long-term memory. Damage can occur to the memory center of the brain, called the hippocampus. This causes a cyclic effect in that the brain loses the ability to submerge the fear reaction and the individual is always operating on high alert. This constant state of fear means the world around the person is wrought with danger and the memories associated with that fear confirm that assessment.

Fight or Flight of Anxiety

Humankind has always had the benefit of survival instincts to answer threats to safety or perils that may manifest. These instincts allow for two responses – flight, as in the running away from danger – or fight – facing an opponent head-on. Humans are not facing the same dangers that plagued prehistoric ancestors. The fight-or-flight response is still active in modern humankind, and it triggers physiological responses in the body in reaction to these perceived threats and dangers, whether these threating scenarios will cause bodily pain or mental anguish. In the case of anxieties and phobias, the dangers are not physical but the psychological reaction to stressors.

These instincts to get away or stay and fight is often referred to as the acute stress response. When this response is activated, the body releases hormones such as adrenaline and cortisol, among others. Other physical symptoms that display with this response an increased blood pressure, pale or flushed skin, dilated pupils and trembling. Once triggered, it could take up to an hour for the body's reactions to dissipate and functions return to normal.

The original intent of these physiological responses was to prepare the body for battle and to heighten awareness of the potential dangers. For example, while in this heightened state, the body's ability to clot blood faster is activated to reduce the loss of blood from injuries. The pupils dilate to help vision improve, and the person can focus on any nearby threats. As the body's muscles tense for the fight, trembling may occur.

While this response in the ancestors was likely triggered by an attack from a saber-tooth tiger or an attack coming from of a competing tribe, today's response may be activated by a growling dog, an annual job performance review from a boss or a sales pitch to win a multi-million-dollar contract. It could also be triggered by less threatening events, such as taking a college entrance exam or even filling out a job application. Fight-or-flight is not only triggered by a physical attack, such as a mugger or rapist, but also by psychological factors.

By priming your body for action, you are better prepared to perform under pressure. The stress created by the situation can actually be helpful, making it more likely that you will cope effectively with the threat. This type of stress can help you perform better in situations where you are under pressure to do well, such as at work or school. In cases where the threat is life-threatening, the fight-or-flight response can play a critical role in your survival. By gearing you up to fight or flee, the fight-or-flight response makes it more likely that you will survive the danger.

The body's responses in the fight or flight are controlled by the nervous system. When confronted with a real threat, such as an angry animal with claws and fangs, its good to know the body has a response to this situation. When confronted by an angry customer, choosing to fight or choosing escape would likely not result in a positive outcome. Learning to control this reaction reduces the amount of stress a person is subjected to. A constant state of stress is harmful to the body's innate defenses.

Understanding the body's reaction to stressful situations and recognizing the signs that the fight-or-flight response is being triggered is essential to learning how to manage stress. The management techniques to calm the physiological and psychological reactions to a real or perceived danger results in a healthier mind and body. Stress management, and with it the ability to calm the fight-or-flight response, is key to resolving physical, emotional and mental health concerns.

Panic Attacks

Panic is defined as a sudden uncontrollable fear or anxiety, often causing wildly unthinking behavior. There are many words to describe this, such as terror, agitation, and hysteria among others. One of the effects of severe anxiety is what health professionals call a panic attack.

It is a common occurrence. An estimated 2.4 million people suffer a panic attack each year in the United States. It usually begins when a person is in their latter part of the teenage years and early young adult stage.

This attack is a period of extreme fear that causes grave reactions by the body as if the body was responding to danger as in the fight or flight response. A person who is experiencing a panic attack may think he or she is having a heart attack, losing control of their physical and mental abilities, or even that death is near. It is a frightening experience for the individual, as well as family members or friends.

Panic attacks can happen once in a while or can be a chronic consequence of an anxiety disorder. It can also trigger another fear that another attack is imminent.

There is no way to predict when a panic attack is going to occur. That complicates the situation for the person who is experiencing it. He or she could be in the middle of an activity, such as driving a vehicle. The attack may occur when he or she is with others or when they are alone.

The sudden onset of a panic attack means there is no way to prevent one from occurring. The attack does not have to be triggered by a stressor of any kind.

Symptoms occurring as the panic attack progresses will peak quickly. The person will feel exhausted and fatigued when the attack dissipates. When the stressful or anxiety causing situation is resolved or removed, the attack will subside.

Look for these most common symptoms to determine if a person is having a panic attack. The person will feel a loss of control and a sense of doom. Their heart rate will increase, they will begin sweating profusely, and likely complain of a headache, chest pain or dizziness.

Panic attacks also involve trembling, numbness or tingling, and abdominal cramping or nausea. Hot flashes are also a common symptom as are the chills.
The good news that panic attacks on their own are not life-threatening, but it is important to seek medical advice to make sure the attacks were anxiety related and not caused by a medical condition.

Social Anxiety and the Mind

Remember the first day at a new school? Or the first day at a new job? How about going to a party at which most of the people are strangers? What happens when it's time to share an opinion on the company's new sales campaign?

All of these examples are situations in which someone who has social anxiety may have a difficult time making it through without a panic attack. Everyone gets nervous about meeting people and standing out in a crowd. Usually, those first meeting jitters give way to more confidence as the meeting and greeting conclude. Those with social anxiety, however, don't see these situations as minor moments of nervousness. For people who have been diagnosed with social anxiety disorder, these happenings are frightening and often unbearable.

Social anxiety is the fear that a person will be judged negatively by others. This fear leads the person to feel inadequate, inferior, self-conscious, embarrassed and humiliated, usually without cause. These self-deprecating thoughts seldom surface when the person is alone, only when in a social or professional setting in which attention may focus on the person.

The situations in which social anxiety may take hold of a person include being introduced to a group of people, having to say something in front of a crowd or a class or boardroom scenario. Social anxiety distress also occurs when those afflicted are teased or criticized, being watched while they do something, or when meeting influential or important people.

Social anxiety disorder, which was previously called social phobia, is estimated to affect millions of people all over the world. In the United States, studies have determined that it is the third most common psychological disorder affecting about seven percent of the population.

Like other anxiety disorders, social anxiety disorder is an extreme reaction to a fear, in this case of social disapproval. Some people have a general type of social anxiety which manifests in almost all types of human interaction, and others have a more specific variation of social anxiety, such as answering questions in class or doing oral presentations.

A person with social anxiety will react to uncomfortable situations with intense fear, and showing signs of physiological distress, including a rapid heart rate, a flushed face, dry mouth, muscle twitches and trembling.

Most people diagnosed with this disorder logically understand that their feelings are not based on fact, but simply their own perceptions. Psychologists explain that understanding that these negative thoughts about what others are thinking about him or her are different than accepting reality. Any social misstep is exaggerated by those with social anxiety, even though it may not have mattered to anyone else.

Myths About Social Anxiety

There are many misconceptions about social anxiety. Like all myths, perpetuating these falsehoods is unfair to those who have to deal with the repercussions of their disorder every day.

- Myth: Social Anxiety is the same as shyness.

It is easy to confuse social anxiety and shyness. People who are shy exhibit many of the same characteristics as those with social anxiety disorder. Shy people are uncomfortable in social situations; they are reluctant to talk to people they don't know and are not likely to voluntarily share their opinions or comments.

Those with social anxiety do not always avoid situations. In fact, anxiety occurs because they are in these situations.

Shyness could be considered a form of social anxiety. Shy people withdraw from social contact and avoid contact with others. The reasons for the shyness could be partly blamed on fear.

- Myth: Fears of public speaking are the only way social anxiety is triggered.

While a requirement to present a dissertation on some academic subject or a speech on economic development may create anxiousness and fear in the presenter, social anxiety is not limited to this narrow scenario.

Social anxiety disorder encompasses a wide range of interpersonal relationships, whether conducted in a professional or casual environment, with strangers or acquaintances. It could be a special occasion, like making a toast at a wedding or it could occur while having dinner out with friends or family.

The type of social encounter or the atmosphere has the same impact. The anxiety is a result of the fear that the person with social anxiety is being judged negatively.

- Myth: There is no solution to social anxiety other than learning to live with it.

Each person who is diagnosed with a social anxiety disorder will have a different experience. Some will have such severe responses to the thought of interacting with people that they seldom leave home or hold down a job. Others interact and be part of the community, but may have a specific fear, such as being in charge or the center of attention or possibly speaking in public.

Those with a social anxiety disorder can be helped with effective treatments. Medication is one option, and another is cognitive-behavioral therapy. With these solutions, a social anxiety disorder can be managed.

- Myth: Social anxiety is just nervousness.

Nervousness is just one of the symptoms of social anxiety disorder. It also involves physiological changes as the anxiety level increases. The capability to think, such as in engaging in small talk, is affected, as is the person's emotions.

The idea of meeting someone new isn't the cause of social anxiety; it's how that person may judge the person with social anxiety.

People are nervous when doing anything for the first time. For those with social anxiety, the distress goes above and beyond the effects of nervousness.

- Myth: Social anxiety disorder does not cause any harm to a person.

Like all forms of stress, social anxiety causes the body to react in physical, emotional and psychological ways. Elevated heart rates, rapid breathing and other physiological consequences that occur chronically can cause other medical conditions.

Stress is a serious consequence and over time can result in premature aging, loss of cognitive functions and serious medical conditions such as heart disease, diabetes, and ulcers.

When Social Anxiety Gets Serious

Unlike training for a marathon or perfecting a musical arrangement, social anxiety disorder does not get easier the more times a person experiences it. In fact, the opposite is true.

Without intervention and a plan of treatment, anxieties can compound and take its toll on work, family and social relationships. Each time social anxiety is triggered, it creates reinforces the fears that the person has about being negatively evaluated.

Continued focus on the perceived negative judgments of others causes low self-esteem, the development of poor social skills, preference for isolation, withdrawal from family and friends, and low achievement. These consequences can also lead to substance abuse and even the taking of one's life.

As social anxiety progresses, it may become increasingly difficult for the person to stay employed or stay connected with friends and family. The isolation that occurs can lead to other disorders, complicating treatment.

Social anxiety is often accompanied by other mental health disorders, such as depression. The possibility of other diagnoses compounds the serious consequences of social anxiety disorder.

It is better to seek help before the disorder becomes too ingrained in the person's lifestyle. When seeking help, provide as much information as possible to the mental health practitioner. This information can be detailed in a journal to help the person, and the practitioner determines what seems to be the predominant stressor in their daily routine.

As social anxiety progresses, it will limit the life experiences available to the person who suffers from the disorder. Pushing past the anxiety will become more difficult, and the maintenance of a normal life becomes almost impossible.

What Is a Phobia?

Everyone has their fears. Some people do not like spiders; others are afraid of snakes. One person may be scared of heights, and another person may become irrational when in the presence of a clown.

When these fears become excessive and irrational, it is called a phobia. People who have a phobia often react in the extreme when they encounter their fear. Whatever it is that triggers this fear, a phobia is specific in nature and revolves around an object, place, or situation.

A fear may cause a nervous feeling in the stomach. A phobia may cause someone to avoid a situation completely. Extreme panic reactions are also common for phobias.

Phobias are a serious disorder because it can affect that individual's daily life. It can stop them from going to work or school, it can intrude upon their personal relationships, and it can alter the way they want to live their lives. Phobias affect about 19 million people in the United States.

The causes of phobias are genetic and environmental. Someone who has experienced a trauma or witnessed a tragic event may develop a phobia. A person who may have suffered an accident in the water can develop aquaphobia. A person who was bitten by a dog in childhood may have cynophobia.

Age, gender and socioeconomic status are also risk factors in developing certain phobias. For example, men are more prone to develop phobias related to medical or dental procedures. Women are more likely to suffer from a fear of animals. Children who grow up in economically challenged households are more likely to be diagnosed with phobias related to social situations.

Phobias may also be triggered by chronic medical conditions or health concerns in general. Those who have experienced a traumatic brain injury, have substance abuse issues or have been diagnosed with depression often develop phobias.

In general, most phobias can be categorized into five distinct areas, according to the Diagnostic and Statistical Manual of Mental Disorders provided by the American Psychiatric Association. These categories are fears related to animals or insects; fears related to the natural environment; fears related to blood, injury, or medical issues; fears related to specific situations; and the "other" category which covers fears that are not related to the other four categories.

Some of the most common phobias are:
- Agoraphobia: a fear of places or situations in which the person feels trapped, such as in a crowded public place
- Acrophobia: the fear of heights
- Arachnophobia: the fear of spiders
- Astraphobia: the fear of thunder and lightning
- Autophobia: the fear of being alone
- Aviophobia: fear of flying.
- Claustrophobia: a fear of enclosed or tight spaces, such as elevators

- Dentophobia: the fear of the dentist or dental procedures.
- Glossophobia: the fear of speaking in front of an audience. It is also known as performance anxiety.
- Hemophobia: a fear of blood or injury
- Mysophobia: the fear of dirt and germs
- Nyctophobia: the fear of nighttime or the dark
- Ophidiophobia: the fear snakes

People who have phobias often experience physiological changes when confronted by what they fear. This can include an accelerated heartbeat, shortness of breath or hyperventilation, speech difficulties, and other symptoms related to panic attacks. In some cases, a person with a phobia may faint or pass out or be unable to move. Others will be moved to tears, and others get aggressive.

A common perception is that a person can overcome their phobias by confronting what it is that they fear. There is some narrative evidence that facing an object of fear can help lessen the reaction of the individual.

A mental health therapy called flooding is designed to place a patient in close proximity to their phobia. This is usually done in combination with other therapies and under the supervision of the therapist. Taking a self-help approach and using the flooding method may make the phobia worse or create a more panicked situation.

If someone responds by fleeing the scene, it could become dangerous because the reaction is to get away from the object that frightens them. If someone strikes out when frightened, others could be injured when that person reacts.

Treating a phobia is best handled by someone who has the training and experience to oversee the treatment. In most cases, it does not take very long to achieve some sort of positive result from treatment. Occasionally medications are also used in combination with therapy.

Learning ways to deal with the fear that a phobia brings on is beneficial. Instead of flooding, another way to build resistance to a phobia is desensitization, which is the gradual exposure to the object of the phobia.

Anxiety, social anxiety, and phobias are serious problems that directly impact the way people live their lives. Therapy and treatment can help reduce the reaction to situations which cause anxiety or fear. While some strategies, such as learning coping skills, can be mastered without professional guidance, it is always recommended that therapy is administered by trained professionals who have the know-how and experience to intervene if needed.

There is no common denominator, no common thread that can identify what situations will cause someone to panic or be overcome with worry and fear. Most of the time, fears are manageable. When they become life-affecting, it is time to seek help.

Chapter 2: Managing Social Anxiety

Hope is powerful, especially to someone for whom the everyday encounter of others is part of a nervous, scary, or even emotional possibility. In addition to the standard treatment offered by mental health professionals, such as therapy and or medications, there are ways for someone with social anxiety to take some level of control back by doing some homework to manage the effects of the disorder.

Part of this management rationale is to change the way the mind thinks and reacts. It is striving to change the way a person sees themselves and the inner dialogue that feeds anxiety.

Managing social anxiety means working on the individual to change the way that they view their abilities. Raising self-confidence and rewiring the brain to replace a negative point of view with a positive one can make a tremendous difference in dealing with the aggravations, fear, and emotional turmoil of anxiety.

Some of the common stressors for a person with social anxiety include public speaking or talking in public, attending parties and galas, conversing with strangers, waiting in line, using public restrooms and public transportation, and doing any activity in front of others.

Rewiring the Thinking Patterns

Social anxiety is triggered by thoughts as opposed to actions, which makes it difficult to avoid. While it is possible to remove oneself from any human interaction, that is not a healthy choice nor is it a lifestyle of value and quality. For the person with social anxiety disorder, it is the thought that he or she is being negatively judged by others, which then ultimately creates the anxiety.

One way to overcome the thoughts associated with a person's feelings of inadequacy that stems from their social anxiety disorder is to change the way the thoughts are perceived and to reinterpret the negative into a positive. Rewiring the negative thoughts with positive ones is a step forward but one that will take perseverance and training.

A daily routine of positive affirmations and challenging perceptions with reality is needed. This is not an easy fix. Unlike reconditioning the human body, reconditioning the mind is much more difficult. As muscles are toned and strengthened, there are obvious results. As changes are made in the thought patterns, people with a social anxiety disorder may not be aware of any progress being made.

One of the first thinking patterns to be challenged is that being anxious is unnatural. Anxiousness is part of the human experience. It is a throwback to the ancestors who only had their instincts to rely on. Anxiousness is the body's way of gearing up for a challenge—and it makes sure that whatever challenge may be ahead, the individual is ready to do their best.

Worrying about how others perceive each other is not uncommon. Everyone is vulnerable to feeling criticized, bullied, ignored or excluded from a group. Human beings are tribal in nature and learned interdependency to survive the trials and tribulations. People are social creatures, and group acceptance and inclusion is important.

It is important to remember that not everyone is going to find universal acceptance by every human being on the planet. People with whom there is much in common are more likely to be accepting of people who are similar themselves. Acceptance of the fact that everyone will, at times in their life, feel the sting of rejection. Accepting this can help ease the impact of those occasions when social anxiety kicks in.

Often these thought patterns are a result of genetics. Research has determined that anxiety is common through generations in a family.

Or, these thought patterns are a result of an environment in which family members were suspicious of those outside their family and social circles. Growing up in an environment in which others were inhospitably treated or were publicly judged in a supercritical and negative manner also sets in motion the idea that this treatment of others is the norm. This thought pattern could also have come from humiliating experiences either as a child or an adult.

Another way to reprocess the thinking that occurs within the mind of someone who experiences social anxiety is to change the way anxiety is perceived. For example, excitement and anticipation of something good happening mirror the same physiological effects as anxiety. People who are in love often have "butterflies" and other physical symptoms that indicate that their body is responding to anxiousness. Instead of a dialogue that focuses on being anxious, substitute excited instead.

Remember that what you think about what will happen is not reality. Human beings have a constant inner dialogue that helps them get through the day. People use these thoughts to determine a course of action to take or what to say when called on in class. These inner conversations can be helpful, but they can also be detrimental, especially for a person with social anxiety.

Instead of using this inner dialogue as reassurance of their abilities, it becomes a voice of worry and fuels any anxiety a person may be feeling. Instead of being an optimistic pep talk about the possibilities, the inner voice of a person with social anxiety disorder is predicting the worst possible outcome. Their inner voice is telling them that people won't like them, that their presentation will be rejected, or their performance publicly criticized.

To change this routine and change the dynamics between what the inner voice expects and the reality of the situation, a person must become more aware of what they are thinking and why this thought is prevailing. A journal or diary can prove helpful in understanding what sparks the negative dialogue and which situations are the most significant in fueling this anxiety.

Record not only the where's and why's about what is causing the anxiety but make an effort to record the thoughts occurring as the situation unfolds. Include any positive outcome, such as a compliment given, or a new acquaintance made, to create a positive memory of the event.

Unlike strategies which use positive thinking as a motivator, when someone with a social anxiety disorder begins looking at the situation realistically, the thought processes behind the anxiety begin to change.

Those afflicted with a social anxiety disorder can also learn to refocus the attention on how to be better prepared for the situation. When a person is anxious, his or her attention is focused on feelings and how their body is responding. Training the person to instead go over notes for a presentation or listening intently to conversations changes the direction of thoughts from inward to outward. Notice the details in the rook or the clothes a person is wearing. This change in focus diverts attention away from fears and anxiety into an awareness of the surroundings.

One technique that has helped change the way in which people with social anxiety disorders look at trigger situations is called Acceptance and Commitment Therapy. This encourages people to face their anxieties, to put up with the nervousness and uncomfortable feelings. With this therapy, clients learn to be aware of their discomfort but forge ahead anyway to keep their lives on track.

Boosting Self-Confidence

A low level of self-confidence is one of the effects that social anxiety disorder causes in a person who suffers from it. Although self-confidence and self-esteem are used interchangeably, these terms refer to very different perceptions. Self-esteem is defined as how a person values themselves. Self-confidence reflects an individual's assurance that in their own abilities to complete tasks, respond to demands and face challenges and their trust in making the right decisions and judgments.

Someone who is afflicted by social anxiety will question whether they have the abilities, talents, skills, knowledge, etc. to handle the social situation well. A student who has practiced for a speech to be given in class has memorized the content but will fear that he or she will not remember the speech, or may not have included the most important information, or that he or she may stumble over the words or mispronounce them.

The fear that somehow their abilities are not enough to protect them from ridicule or criticism is what drives social anxiety. Building confidence can quiet these fears and although the person who has a social anxiety disorder may still experience discomfort, boosting self-confidence can provide encouragement to follow through with the experience or opportunity.

Belief is one's abilities, skills, and talents make it easier to experience new things, to put one's self in situations that may be uncomfortable. It keeps a person moving forward in life, such as deciding to change careers, ask for a promotion, begin dating, or hosting a holiday party. For a person with social anxiety, these situations are fraught with fear, but improving this person's self-confidence can impact their abilities to follow through.

To improve one's belief in their abilities, there are some tips that can help.

- Don't compare yourself to others: When a person compares themselves to another person, that comparison is often based on external factors, such as occupation, annual salary, college degree, etc. Those who make these comparisons are likely to become envious of what another person has. According to research, there is a correlation between envy and a person's perceptions of themselves. Comparisons do not take into account the personal struggles, sacrifices, efforts or circumstances it took for someone to get to a particular point in their life. Assuming that everyone's

path is the same is not only erroneous but detrimental to self-confidence.
- Build your confidence by putting yourself in the situations that cause you anxiety, even if it's only by role-playing with trusted friends. Ask a stranger how to get to the grocery store, introduce yourself to a fellow parent at your child's school. Each time a person makes it through these scenarios, confidence builds.
- Look for positive outcomes in every situation you experience. Acknowledge the applause you receive, respond to genuine greetings, note the smiles from people you encounter. Tallying these positive affirmations reinforces positive experiences and builds confidence that similar responses will accompany other experiences.
- Treat yourself with kindness. When a mistake is made, or something does not go as planned, consider that no one is perfect. Mistakes happen all the time to everyone. Instead of chastising yourself, roleplay how you would comfort a friend who had messed up.
- Jump in despite your doubts. When someone is unsure of how well they will do, they often forego trying. That leaves talents untapped, such as a closet singer who would be awesome in a community theater's performance of My Fair Lady or an artist's innovative technique that stays hidden from public exhibition. Prepare for the opportunity, whether that means memorizing a speech or getting better at small talk. Try out your talents in front of family and friends and practice to build confidence.
- A healthy body is a confidence builder. Eating properly, getting plenty of sleep and engaging in physical activity benefit the body and the mind. Getting exercise and staying healthy provides a positive outlook.

Managing Self-Consciousness

Self-Consciousness is simply being aware of one's self, especially to have a heightened awareness. This awareness often makes a person uncomfortable because of the perceptions a person has about themselves and how he or she believes others will see them.

Ever been called on to answer a question in class? When this happens, a person will become nervous. Instead of focusing on the answer, that person may instead be focusing on how their body is responding to being called on. Perhaps he or she begins sweating. Maybe their face gets flushed. When the focus shifts from an external point of view to an internal one, that is self-consciousness in action.

The problem with this is that for someone with a social anxiety disorder, this self-awareness often comes with negative thoughts. The person may lose focus on the question or the task and instead worry about how those around them will judge their nervousness. It can result in acting out of character or responding in a way that would not normally be an option without the onset of self-consciousness.

Self-consciousness is influenced not only be a person's own insecurities but by societal pressures as well. It no longer is simply something that happens in a face-to-face situation, but it can also occur during interaction on social media or in an online environment. Because of technology and digital access, there is no place that is safe for a person who has a social anxiety disorder. The pressure to fit into this often self-centered and narcissistic social media world is tough when a person is preoccupied with how others perceive them.

Self-consciousness is best illustrated as the voices in a person's head that repeat the negative perceptions the person has collected through their years. The insecurities, the hurt feelings, the playground comments from bullies all take a toll. These comments are stored in the memory, and when a person is experiencing self-consciousness, these memories are replayed. "You're weird. You're ugly. People are laughing at you. Don't embarrass yourself."

The list goes on and acts to remind the person of all the perceived failings in life. When self-consciousness kicks in, the fear of eliciting that same response surfaces. A person who was rejected when asking someone out on a date may carry that rejection with them, affecting their ability to ask another person out. Someone who was teased because of the way they pronounced a word, will be reluctant to speak in public. Because a person is aware of these perceptions, self-consciousness could make them respond differently in situations. Someone who is outgoing may become more introverted. A person may try harder to impress people when he or she is seeking acceptance by a group. Blending in instead of standing out may be the only option for someone whose self-consciousness is elevated.

Comments made by others about another person are not necessarily reality. But it is difficult to silence these harsh critics when a person has a high-level response to self-consciousness. The tendency to act natural or be ourselves is pushed aside; instead, a person reacts in the way they believe will shield them from criticism.

To combat the influence of this negative inner voice, a person has to identify what is damaging about these perceptions as well as how this perception became so ingrained in the mind.

Once this understanding is realized, there are steps to take that can help a person overcome this destructive self-conscious state.

- Challenge self-criticism, the first step, requires the individual to identify the source of the criticism and counter the criticism with a reality-based viewpoint that is kinder and more compassionate. It calls for the development of awareness – how these inner criticisms influence a person's behavior and reactions and how this criticism detracts from the person's goals and accomplishments.

- Cut yourself some slack: Becoming your own best friend is good advice to move on past the self-consciousness. What do you admire about your friends? What are their good qualities? Take these reflections and turn the light on yourself. Learning to appreciate the individual traits, strengths, and uniqueness about ourselves is a way to counter the negative perceptions a person has stored away. Replace those critiques with self-compliments.

- Do a reality check in your head: An individual's actions, behavior, personality or appearance is always more important to themselves than to others. People who are self-conscious inflate the negative reactions they perceive about themselves and project this same reaction to those around them.

For example, a department supervisor is asked to lead a training session for his or her employees. The presentation involves policy and procedures which the department head has formulated, with the approval of management. As the presentation begins, the supervisor makes a mistake. He or she quickly catches it but has a hard time getting over the embarrassment of making a mistake in front of staff. Internally, the supervisor is thinking that the employees are smirking at his or her discomfort. The voice inside the supervisor's head may say, "You don't know what you're doing, and now everyone knows." In reality, the staff is probably not paying close attention to the presentation or have formed no opinion. In reality, most people know how difficult it is to speak in front of others and are likely glad they were not the ones who had to give this presentation.

- Lighten your mood: Remember that everyone makes mistakes and finding the humor in something that did not go as planned takes the pressure off helps a person move on. Very few mistakes or errors are as serious as a person thinks and making a joke or funny comment tips the scales toward a healthy balance.

Find strength in who you are: In the laws of physics, every action has an equal and opposite reaction. When a person steps into the spotlight, it is an act of courage. It makes that person vulnerable to feeling unworthy or judged. The vulnerability is a necessary part of finding the strengths of a person. Reading the definition of vulnerability - the quality or state of being exposed to the possibility of being attacked or harmed, either physically or emotionally – makes one question why being vulnerable is something that should be embraced to build a better self-image. Don't we want to protect ourselves from harm and attacks? Isn't that what made us doubt our abilities in the first place?

If a person weren't open to experiencing new things, that person would not become aware of what their ambitions are, what ignites the passion, and what motivates them. Experiencing new things, meeting new people, going to places never visited opens up the world and allows people to step through. Every time someone quells their fears to step into the spotlight, to be social, to put a hand out to make an acquaintance, it builds confidence. The person learns that not every foray into new territory is a negative experience.

When an individual learns who they are, they replace vulnerability with strength. Each time fears give way to courage a person finds something they do well. Setbacks, such as the negative thoughts planted in the mind by others, take extra effort to overcome. Finding out more about the individual is that extra effort to transplant the negative judgments with positive, self-affirming ones.

Practice turning negative judgments about yourself into positive ones: With a slight change in words, a negative statement can become an inspirational one. Simply making a better word choice or correcting a negative statement when it is made can start the process of what's referred to as positive self-talk.

Here are some examples of how this works. Instead of saying "I can't do this," replace that with "I'll do the best I can." Instead of "Everything is going wrong" say "One step at a time and I will handle this." Instead of saying "I'll probably make a mistake," focus on what you have done to prepare.

This technique is not something that you have to use only when anxiety kicks in. By practicing turning negative statements into positive ones, it will become second nature.

Chapter 3: Social Anxiety in Daily Life

Going to work, going to school, grocery shopping, running errands, attending a teacher-parent conference at your children's school, heading to the gym, meeting friends for dinner, and going to the movies—these are all activities that a person may do as part of their daily life. The activities are familiar ones that are done as part of a routine, at familiar locations. No problem, right?

For someone with a social anxiety disorder, any or all of these routine tasks could be debilitating and fear-inducing. Everyday life for someone who is afflicted with social anxiety disorder is not routine. There is fear about going to the wrong door at your daughter's school—anxiety that your plan to reorganize the department is not going to win the boss' approval.

Social anxiety revolving around everyday tasks causes people to withdraw. It takes people out of the world and into self-imposed isolation. Their daily life is filled with worry and self-doubt, apprehension and avoidance, and defensive posturing. All of these negative emotions zap the joy out of being an active part of the community. Instead, the person with social anxiety travels through their day—hoping he or she won't be noticed, that he or she can simply blend in.

This scenario is much more common than most people believe. In the United States, social anxiety disorder is the third most diagnosed mental health concern.

A person with social anxiety will walk through the neighborhood in fear that people are watching him or her. In the socially anxious mind, people are judging them for what they are doing wrong. Maybe their shoes don't match their suit—or maybe people will think they walk funny.

A simple task like going to the bank is fear-inducing because it means being in the presence of other people, having to answer a pleasant greeting, or not knowing what to say or how to respond when someone engages in friendly conversation. What if he or she filled the deposit slip out incorrectly? What if he or she stammers when telling the teller what they want? What if they can't figure out how to send the drive-thru container back to the teller? What judgments will others make about them?

Meeting friends for a relaxing dinner is not possible for social anxiety. There will be people they don't know in the restaurant. Even though they are with people they know, it is the opinions of those they don't know that will cause anxiety. What if he or she drops a fork and everyone looks at them? What if he or she mispronounces the name of the entrée? What if they laugh too loudly?

Someone with social anxiety will avoid making a phone call, opting instead to pay a bill online or without the need for human interaction. Without having to talk to someone, he or she protects their psyche from the negative judgments they are sure will come from a human-to-human conversation. Perhaps the customer service associate will judge him or her for not speaking clearly—or for misreading their 13-digit account number.

When it comes to interacting with someone in charge, such as a boss, a teacher, a police officer, etc., people with social anxiety often react more severely. Anyone who he or she would consider to be "better" in some way will cause the symptoms of anxiety to manifest, such as an increased heart rate, sweatiness, a flushed face, or conversely, a paling of the face. It's similar to being sent to the principal's office as a child, the feeling of fear that a person is in trouble for something they said or did.

There are techniques and helpful suggestions to help those with social anxiety get through the day. There are also therapies that are helpful in helping those with this disorder manage their anxiety.

Keeping the Mind Calm

An important technique that helps those with social anxiety is to find ways to calm the mind from the nervousness and anxiety that builds in socially stressful situations. Achieving a quiet and relaxed state of mind can counter the effects of anxiety. Practicing techniques regularly as part of a daily ritual helps prolong the calming effect these have on the mind.

Several techniques work on the theory of mindfulness, a type of meditation that connects people with their thoughts and impressions. Acceptance of anxiety is a key component in using mindfulness as a resource to overcome the source of social anxiety. Knowing that the person's thoughts and feelings are wrapped up in the anxiety and accepting that is a difficult, but essential step in the process.

Waging war between the calm of mindfulness and the fury of anxiety does not achieve any long-lasting benefits. It doesn't provide any quick or short-term relief either. Mindfulness is a process of becoming aware of your thoughts, your physiological reactions and using conscious acknowledgment and affirmations to negate the effects of the anxious mind.

For mindfulness to be effective, the person has to practice the techniques without any expectations of change. Mindfulness is not a cure for social anxiety; it is simply a way of calming down the impact of the negative thoughts. It is also understanding that the body may be restless, the mind may wander, and thoughts. Mindfulness is about paying attention to what is happening and taking care to follow through with the breathing and meditation exercises each time. It is being mindful of what your mind and body are doing and experiencing at that moment in time, not 10, 20, 30 minutes before or even a week or month ago. It is in the present, right now.

Mindfulness is designed to give the individual the power to observe their own thoughts and process these in a way that resonates. Are the thoughts that come into a mind like fish in a stream, swimming into view and swimming out of view? Are these thoughts like clouds that drift across the sky? By practicing mindfulness, the person notices patterns in how he or she responds to thoughts, why some thoughts are given more importance than others and which thoughts draw interest.

Other ways to achieve a calmer mind use cognitive therapies to change the way a person interacts with the thoughts that occur.

- Separate your identity from your thoughts: Cognitive Defusion is a type of therapy that asks the person undergoing this technique to view their thoughts as information but not as a reflection of themselves. When someone is anxious, the thoughts that occur are the result of the mind's flight or fight response. The nervousness and anxiety are a result of how the brain is communicating anticipation of danger or harm. Thoughts that accompany this response are simply words and images.

Cognitive defusion tells the anxious mind that it has a choice: it can validate or not validate the thoughts that surround social anxiety. Having a choice means the person can choose to dismiss the negative thoughts in favor of finding a solution that works for them. Thoughts are a barrier to moving on. Cognitive defusion lessens the importance of these thoughts as it applies to the individual.

- Put your thoughts into categories without bothering with the content: The advantage of this mental exercise is to allow the mind to focus on the type of thoughts that are constructive as opposed to destructive. Some thoughts require a judgment; some are based on worry; others are based on hopes, and others are based on fond memories. Why waste effort on dealing with judgmental thoughts or worrisome ones?

Categorizing the type of thoughts allows the mind to skip over those that may be anxiety-producing in favor of ones that are neutral as far as the mind is concerned.

- Time changes all things: Many of the negative thoughts a person with a social anxiety disorder has come from past unpleasant experiences. Learning to dwell in the present distances the person from remembering the person, place or event that contributed to the development of their social anxiety. That time when he failed that test in fourth grade and disappointed his parents – that was a long time ago before he graduated with honors from high school and college. Remembering that embarrassing fourth-grade test disaster may be one of the sources for his anxiety when it comes to being tested, graded, or reviewed today.

By reiterating that a person is not the same as they were in the past, that situations faced as an adult are not the same as those they faced as a child, that the people we encounter when we have free choice as to whom we wish to associate is different than when we were forced into study groups in school. Change is not necessarily a bad thing and realizing that the changes a person has undergone have shaped them and given them perspective. How has your life experience as an adult made you better able to cope with adversity?

- Discern helpful facts from unhelpful ones: When a person looks at a situation and analyzes the facts, sometimes they focus on the one that feeds into their doubts and fears. For example, a student applying to a prestigious college may focus on the fact that only 20 percent of those that apply are selected. Thinking that he or she has a four out of five chance of making the cut is defeating. By dismissing this fact, that student can focus on completing the application requirements to present themselves in the best possible light.

Calming the mind takes an approach that addresses the validity of the thoughts that surface when a person is anxious or nervous. Calming the mind also means calming the inner dialogue and teaching the brain to use logic and reason to analyze the thought process revolving around anxiety.

Managing Anxious Thoughts

Exercises to calm the mind are a good tool to have in working towards a reduction in the effects of social anxiety. But what can be used when a person is in the middle of an anxiety episode? Thoughts related to a person's social anxiety come fast, intense and recurring. These thought patterns happen whenever anxiety or stress is present, even if none of the other symptoms manifest.

Most of the time these inner beliefs are reminders of the past, of a similar time when these same feelings surfaced, such as a time of sadness, loss, or embarrassment. But, the possibilities of what will happen in the future can also be triggered. There is no pattern to these thought patterns, but they are usually overinflated worries.

It is tough and tiring to deal with these thought patterns, especially since the thoughts come quickly when the mind is agitated. It's like the brain is running on a treadmill and cannot get off. It's more difficult to focus and effects a person's ability to complete chores and even to sleep.

Slowing down the anxious mind takes a little effort but can easily be accomplished.

- Change how you view anxious thoughts: There is no use trying to avoid anxious thoughts. Repression does not work. Instead, change the way you process these. The act of reframing these thoughts as guesses reduces their importance. When the mind considers something as a fact, it suggests that the outcome is already assured. Facts are seldom wrong, but guesses are right only some of the time, depending on the odds. Counter the negative predictions of what could happen by looking at the other side of the coin. What good can come from the situation? Use your experience to determine the most likely outcome based on what you know as fact.

This technique is called cognitive distancing. Simply put, this means that understanding a situation has to take place via several points of view. Scenarios have to be looked at, and outcomes have to be weighed, both negative and positive as well as a combination of both.

- Find a calming phrase: Adopting a mantra is a proven technique to quiet the mind in a stressful situation. According to studies, the repetition of a mantra activates the area of the brain in which self-judgment and reflection occur.

There's no science to picking out a sound, word, or phrase that will act as a mantra. It simply has to be something that will allow you to focus on the mantra instead of anxious thoughts. A favorite positive quote, saying "All is OK," or simply making a sound will work. The key is to use the same mantra every time. Practice ensures that the mantra is committed to memory and can be recalled easily when needed. Don't wait until anxiety happens to practice; make perfecting your mantra recall a daily task.

Reinforcing this mantra with a physical action, like tapping an arm, hand or leg, is also helpful in redirecting the mind away from the anxiety-caused thoughts.
- Document your apprehensions: When in the middle of a stream of anxiety-related thoughts, taking time to write down the fears and dreads allows the person the opportunity to review these concerns later. It also slows

down the continual influx of anxiety-related thoughts, in essence giving the brain a chance to slow down.

There is an order to writing thoughts down because it provides a way to organize and analyze. The time it takes to finish this task calms the mind and diminishes the frenzy of the anxiety-related thoughts. A calmer approach to the fears opens up the door to better reactions.

- Take a break and change the scenery: When the mind continues to focus on the same anxious thoughts, it leaves little opportunity for finding a solution to the dilemma. Standing up, stretching the body, moving to another area, or focusing on a task or activity changes a person's perspective.

An author who is struggling with writer's block may abandon his or her story for a half-hour, an hour or even a day or two. The time away from work allows the author to see things differently. It is easier to spot errors and to find a new approach to the part of the story that was proving difficult.

When someone is having anxious thoughts, turning around or moving to another area can have the same effect. A change in scenery changes the focus and provides perspective.

- Ditch the telephoto view: When a person is experiencing distress because of anxiety, the focus is on the stressor. Limiting the focus on what is causing the anxiety feeds that nervousness. The mind wants to focus on the perceived threat instead of on the complete picture.

Taking a step back to consider more than what is activating the anxiety slows down the rapid rehashing of worry and fear. Just like looking through a microscope, things look bigger than they are in real life. This holds true in reference to anxious thoughts. Giving too much importance to the anxiety makes the person miss other details about the experience.

Managing the Panic Mind

When someone is in the throes of a panic attack, there are various techniques that can be used to counter the physical effects. But what about the mind? How does someone stop the panic from affecting their thoughts and bringing about a calmer demeanor?

In addition to the worry caused by the reaction to the anxiety, during a panic attack, the mind's reaction is to add more fear and doubt. The symptoms of a panic attack mirror those of a heart attack, so one of the worries experienced by those who are having a panic attack is if they are going to die.

Because the thoughts race into the mind so quickly in this situation, finding a way to distract the mind by focusing on something else is one suggestion that helps slow down the thoughts, however, a panic attack is fear multiplied by 10. The instinct is to fight the rollercoaster of thoughts and to force the mind to focus on something else.

Instead, experts advise to wait it out. Let the thoughts race but consider it to be like a wave. During childbirth, women will experience pain in waves based on their contractions. Some of these sensations are strong and almost intolerable, and others cause discomfort. Natural childbirth classes teach techniques that help mothers make it through the toughest parts of the birthing process.

Looking at the waves of thoughts that flood the mind during a panic attack as simply a wave on the beach helps alleviate further panic.

Waves on the shore come in a regular flow, although some are bigger and others smaller. Let your mind experience the thoughts with the reassurance that it will pass.

Distract the mind with the sense of touch. Holding an ice cube in one hand and the other takes the mind's focus off the anxious thoughts. It forces the mind to settle on something in the real world instead of inside the brain. The coldness and irritation from the ice cube snap the brain from panicked thoughts to focus on the discomfort.

Thoughts can also be distracted by doing an activity that requires physical movement or the use of higher brain skills, such as solving a Sudoku puzzle or folding laundry. Because the mind has to concentrate on a task, there is less room to process negative thoughts.

Utilize reason and logic to provide alternative thoughts. Panic attacks originate with the emotions. Reason and logic come from a different part of the brain. Because anxiety and panic are so frightening, it's as if the emotions take control and every other brain functions take a back seat.

Finding a way to engage reason and logic takes control back from the emotions. It redistributes brain power across the whole spectrum instead of focusing exclusively on fear and worry.

Overcoming Panic Attacks

The sudden onset of a panic attack can be frightening. Both the body and the mind are affected when these attacks happen, which can be at any time, even while asleep.

Common symptoms include a fast heart rate, breathing difficulties, a sense of terror, a faint or dizzy feeling, chest pains, tingling or numbness in fingers and hands, sweating or chilled, and an overall feeling that the person has lost control. Panic attacks do not last a long time – most are over in 10 minutes – but it does take longer to recover from some of the symptoms.

Much of the focus on overcoming some of the symptoms of a panic attack involves getting the body to slow down its reactions. Proper breathing techniques in the height of the panic attack are an essential skill that can be used to quell anxiety and minimize stress. Those having a panic attack frequently say it is difficult to catch their breath. Common complaints from those having an attack liken it to a sense of choking, smothering or suffocating.

When a person complains that they are unable to catch their breath, it means they are not getting enough air. During a panic attack, breaths become faster, but the quality of the breathing is shallow. This means that not enough oxygen is being taken into the body and, conversely, too much carbon dioxide is being exhaled. The body needs to maintain a steady level of carbon dioxide to avoid symptoms such as a dry mouth, numbness or tingling, and chest pain caused by the tightening of the chest muscles.

This shortness of breath is also called hyperventilation and is characterized by short, shallow breaths. The danger of hyperventilation is that it can lead to faintness, light-headedness, and confusion.

A sign of someone who may be hyperventilating is the taking of short, quick breaths. Others may cough or exhibit rapid breathing.

The first step is to calm down. Not being able to breathe properly is a scary experience and is likely to cause additional panic.

Experts recommend that a person take slow and deep breaths to ease anxiety. The key to deep breathing is to remember to inhale and exhale at the same pace. To help regulate your breathing, pretend that you are blowing up a balloon.

This is a skill that can be practiced, as the ideal breath should come from the abdomen. Breathe in through the nose for a count of four and then breathe out to the same four-count rhythm. When done correctly, the abdomen should rise, and the chest should remain still.

An alternative to deep breathing is to breathe at a slower pace than your body wants to. During a panic attack, taking breaths at a slower pace puts you in better control of your breathing, and it slows down the heart. This technique is a calming influence on the flight-or-fight response.

As you breathe during a panic attack, parts of the body may tense up. Areas that are most prone to that happening are the jaw, lips, and shoulders. Try relaxing these muscles and see if the breathing improves.

Managing Stress Levels

Everyone, not just those with a social anxiety order or another phobia, has to deal with stress. Stress management is an important health concern. It affects the mind and the body and can lead to serious health issues.

Some stress is easier to handle, as the hassles of traffic jams or an extra tight deadline at the office. Other interactions, like the illness of a family member, the loss of a job, or the death of a loved one add enormous amounts of stress to the usual load.

For someone with social anxiety, managing stress becomes increasingly important to offset the times when the disorder becomes triggered, or in the case of a panic attack.

To expand on the helpfulness of a breathing technique like the one used to minimize the effects of hyperventilation during a panic attack can be especially useful. When linked to another stress reduction method, meditation, the combination has proven to be successful at calming and relaxing the body and mind.

Guided relaxations, meditation, and yoga all use variations of breathing techniques to regulate how the practitioner breaths. In all of these three programs, the goal is to become aware of the body and its functions, including how to draw a breath and how to use this natural and essential bodily function to reduce stress.

Meditation does not have to be an elaborate process. It could involve writing in a journal, indulging in art, even taking up the popular coloring books for adults. While you are involved in any activity that helps you relax and stem the constant flow of worrisome thoughts, focus on the task. It can also be a time to repeat positive, uplifting messages.

There are also scenarios that can help put the brain in the right state of mind. Remembering a special place in a person's life that has happy or relaxing memories is a way to personalize the stress management ritual.

Others may envision their stress triggers moving like the wind in all of its incarnations – a breeze, a gust, a blustery force, or even a storm. Whatever the wind does, the practitioner lets it happen in their mind, holding on to the knowledge that their calmness protects against the unpredictability.

Visualizing being at the ocean is also a common meditation scenario. In this example, the body is caressed by the sun and the sea, and tranquility comes from the rhythmic lull of the waves on the shore. Drawing parallels between the sea and one's life add another dimension to the meditation, serving as an illustrative mechanism to take charge and embrace change.

No matter the relaxation scenario a person chooses, meditation is more than simply imagining yourself in that place. It is about making observations about your meditation spot and determining how the symbolism relates to you. Meditation is learning to delve deeper into our minds and bodies to reduce worry and find inner peace. A peaceful person is happier, healthier and more resistant to stress.

Getting active is another way to reduce stress. A routine visit to the gym, a hike in the woods, or a jog around the park are all activities that produce endorphins to counteract those hormones released during stressful times.

In this technologically connected world, there are options to help people keep track of vitals like heart rate, pulse rate, oxygen levels, and calories expended. These apps are helpful for those who want to keep track of their progress.

Experts suggest several ways to stop stress quickly. These suggestions can be used individually or combined as needed.

- Take time to make a decision about something that is troubling you.
- Recite the alphabet or count to 10 before responding
- Go for a short walk away from the event, the person, or the situation that is causing you to worry.
- Listen to your favorite music, pick up your favorite book or indulge in your passion.
- Spend time with your family, friends, children or pets.
- Dissect a problem into steps and handle one at a time.

Stress Inoculation Training – A Treatment for Social Anxiety

Stress often takes a person without notice. The boss makes significant changes to the internal memo two hours before it is scheduled to be distributed. A parent gets a call that their child suffered an injury during an athletic competition. These are situations which cannot be planned, and the uncertainty is what makes it stressful.

Stress Inoculation Therapy (SIT) is a way of preparing for stressful situations beforehand by training the brain how to react when stress and anxiety occurs. Relaxation and breathing exercise play a role. Those involved in SIT learn to seek a private place to diffuse the anxiety by using coping thoughts. These abilities come from learning about stress and situations which cause stress and crafting the steps they need to take to counteract the negative effects.

For those who have a social anxiety disorder, SIT develops a plan to follow when social anxiety begins to manifest. This plan is developed by anticipating what situations cause the anxiety as well as how the individual typically responds.

SIT's philosophy is that by training a person to anticipate the consequences of a situation that person is "inoculated," or protected to a certain extent from the results of enduring the stressful situation or the social anxiety. A repercussion of repeated exposure to high-stress situations is post-traumatic stress disorder.

SIT has three phases. The first is the conceptual phase. In this phase, the person learns the basics of stress - what it is, how it happens and how it can affect the person. It also delves into how some techniques can have a negative effect when used to manage stress and reinforces effective coping skills. It is in this phase that the person will chart the stressors and how they respond to these. This information is used to fine tune the coping ideas for the individual.

The beginning stages of SIT is used to identify ongoing stressors, something that happens on a regular basis, or a time-limited stressor like a court appearance for a divorce. Every person will have their own list of stressful situations that can benefit from SIT. The training is adaptive to the individual.

The next phase is the skills acquisition and consolidation phase. During this phase, the individual is taught stress management skills developed for the individual according to their plan. These skills include cognitive restructuring, problem-solving, relaxation training, and emotional self-regulation. With these new skills, when the individual is faced with a stressful situation, he or she has options in how to respond.

Finally, the individual enters the application and follow-through phase. This is the time when the skills are put to the test, and the person faces escalating stressors, also known as systematic desensitization. By training the person to become more equipped to handle stressful situations, SIT builds confidence. The person has better self-control and enhances their abilities to reduce the harmful effects of stress.

Chapter 4: Understanding Depression

Depression is a misunderstood mental health issue. Most people equate depression with feeling sad, but it is a lot more than simply being sad, which is a real emotion that everyone experiences from time to time.

Depression goes beyond emotion. It is recognized as an illness by health experts, and every person's bout with depression is not the same as someone else's. There are treatments for depression.

There are several disorders that are classified as a type of depression.

Severe symptoms that cause the person to be unable to work, sleep, eat, or do other ordinary lifestyle tasks is characteristic of major depression. This type of depression can occur multiple times.

A persistent depressive disorder is used to classify a depression with a minimum of two-year duration. The person diagnosed with this disorder is likely to have a combination of major depressive incidents as well as periodic symptoms.

Psychotic depression is a depression that is combined with another psychosis, such as delusions or hallucinations.

Postpartum depression afflicts new mothers. An estimated 10 to 15 percent of women who give birth experience the hormonal and physical effects of this type of depression.

Some people are acutely affected by the seasons, with depression manifesting in the wintertime. This form of depression is called Seasonal Affective Disorder and is triggered by a lack of natural sunlight. Symptoms usually go away in spring. According to statistics, five percent of the population in the United States has seasonal affective disorders—with women making up 80 percent of these diagnoses.

According to statistics, women are more likely to be diagnosed with depression. Likely due, in part, to postpartum depression, women tend to have symptoms relating to sadness, feeling guilty, and worthlessness. Men, on the other hand, are more likely to have symptoms related to fatigue, difficulty sleeping, and loss of interest in activities they once enjoyed.

Children can develop depression in their pre-pubescent years—with occurrences equally distributed between boys and girls. Teens and young adults who show one or more symptoms of depression should be checked out by medical and mental health practitioners. Teenage years are difficult, and stress from school demands and peer influences are higher than at other ages. A child or teen who has been diagnosed with depression will continue to be afflicted into their adult years.

According to statistics compiled by the World Health Organization, an estimated 300 million people worldwide are afflicted with depression. In the United States, 16.2 million adults or 6.7 percent of the population have experienced a problem with depression within a 12-month period.

What Is Depression?

Depression is a life-changing illness that takes its toll on how people live their lives and interact with others. Clinical depression is the official name for the disorder that can show up in a multitude of symptoms.

A person who is depressed creates a difficult dynamic for family and friends. Not only does the depressed person feel the stress of the disorder, but their condition adds stress to family members, too. To offset this, family members are encouraged to take an active role in the diagnosis and treatment of their loved one. Counseling or therapy for the family is also an option.

As an illness, depression requires treatment. It is not something that will cure itself with the passage of time, nor can someone make themselves get better simply by willing it to be so.

Although the symptoms vary, there are some indicators that a person may be suffering from depression. If the signs do not go away in two weeks, health experts suggest that the person may be clinically depressed.

It is important to note that not everyone experiences the same symptoms or combinations of symptoms. People who are diagnosed with depression may experience different levels of severity. For one person, difficulty concentrating may be very severe, and in another, the severest symptom may be appetite changes. Some people struggle with more than a few symptoms, and others experience multiple symptoms.

These signs and symptoms include:

- Persistent sad, anxious, or "empty" mood
- Feelings of guilt, worthlessness, helplessness
- Feelings of hopelessness, pessimism
- Difficulty concentrating, remembering, making decisions
- Decreased energy, fatigue, being "slowed down"
- Difficulty sleeping, early-morning awakening, or oversleeping
- Appetite and/or weight changes
- Restlessness, irritability
- Loss of interest or pleasure in hobbies and activities
- Persistent physical symptoms
- Thoughts of death or suicide, suicide attempts

One particular group of people who are susceptible to developing depression are the elderly. This group presents a challenge because many of the symptoms of depression in younger people are different from those that manifest in older people. Medical diagnoses and prescription side effects are also considerations when determining whether a senior citizen is dealing with depression.

Common symptoms for this age group include feeling tired, being grumpy or irritable. They may have difficulty going to sleep. Confusion is another common symptom, which is also indicative of Alzheimer's Disease, which complicates diagnoses.

On important fact about depression is that it can be treated. As with many disorders, early detection and intervention achieve better results. Medication and therapy are the most common treatment methods, either individually or in combination.

There are many misconceptions about depression that continue to add a stigma to discussions about the disorder. Depression is not sadness nor is it considered a weakness of some kind. It is a diagnosable condition with symptoms and conventional treatment options. It is caused by genetic, biological and psychological factors.

Someone who has depression cannot will themselves out of it. There is no switch that turns it on or turns it off. Changing attitudes or flooding your environment with cheerful thoughts and happy unicorns and rainbows is not a treatment. It has very little to do with grief or sadness and more to do with physiological and psychological reasons.

A tragic incident by itself does not cause depression. Grief over the death of a loved one or the ending of a relationship puts someone at risk of developing depression, but a single incident is not the cause. Depression can manifest when times are good or when times are tough, and it can be part of an ongoing period of lost hope, being withdrawn or loss of interest. Suicide is also a possibility during a depression.

How is it formed?

Like many mental illnesses, depression can be caused by a number of factors.

Genetics is one of the factors that can determine whether a person is at risk for depression. An individual who has family members diagnosed with depression is more likely to develop the disorder as well.

The genes that are part of the makeup of every human being have an effect on mood and personality. If there is a malfunction in the genes, it can change the way people respond, including affecting mood. When the genes are not on target as far as mood is concerned, any situation, event or inconvenience may trigger anxiety and stress.

Brain chemistry and other factors relating to the way the brain functions are also linked to the onset of depression. Research suggests that the chemicals inside the brain of those with depression work differently than that of non-depressed individuals. Hormone imbalances also can lead to depression. Most vulnerable to a hormone-related cause of depression are women who are undergoing a pregnancy or entering menopause.

While a direct correlation between brain chemistry and depression has yet to be formalized, research notes that there is a connection between changes in the brain and the onset of depression. Whether those changes are a result of faulty synapses or caused by elevated levels of hormones produced in stressful situations, a cause of depression is likely linked to the brain.

Trauma, grief or stress are just some of the environmental and life-experience related reasons that depression can manifest. Research also indicates that depression related to trauma does not have to have happened directly to the person that has depression. A person who witnesses tragedy can also become depressed because of it.

Seeing an event unfold such as the terrorist attack on the Twin Towers in New York on 9/11 or school shootings often shatter preconceived notions about how the world works, according to psychologists. This can lead to a panic disorder, which can develop into depression.

Depression begins most often in a person's teenage years into their 20s and 30s. High levels of anxiety in childhood have also been shown to possibly lead to depression later in life.

When depression happens alongside other serious medical diagnoses, such as cancer or Parkinson's disease, it can make conditions worse. Part of the reason this occurs can be linked to the medications used to treat these diseases, a side effect of the prescription drugs.

Depression in the Mind

Depression is a mental health disorder, and the effects of it are related to how the disorder affects brain function. The levels of cortisol, which is regulated by parts of the brain, are indicative of the brain's role in the onset of depression. As an example of this connection, researchers found that the cortisol levels for someone with depression remain high throughout the day as compared to a non-depressed person. Normal brain function records the highest levels of cortisol in the morning and decreases at night.

Science has identified three areas of the brain that are most likely involved in depression. These three have been identified as the hippocampus, amygdala and the prefrontal cortex.

The hippocampus is the memory center of the brain. Located near the center of the brain, one of its primary functions is to produce cortisol. This hormone is released when the flight-or-fight response is activated or simply in times of stress, whether that stress is physical or mental related, and when a person is suffering from depression.

While this hormone is essential as a mechanism to cope with stress when there is too much cortisol produced during stressful events or because of a chemical imbalance, are sent to the brain due to a stressful event or a chemical imbalance in the body. These high levels impact the hippocampus' ability to generate new brain cells. When someone with depression has high levels of cortisol, memory problems are a possibility.

At the front of the brain is the prefrontal cortex. This area of the brain is affected by high levels of cortisol, impacting its abilities to regulate emotions, form memories and assist in a person's decision-making abilities. Too much cortisol has been shown to shrink the prefrontal cortex.

The third part of the brain, the amygdala becomes enlarged when a person has depression due to the high levels of cortisol produced in the hippocampus. The function of this area of the brain is to prompt the appropriate emotional response, such as fear, feelings of happiness or pleasure. When this area of the brain is impacted, sleep will be disrupted, and the usual activity patterns of the individual will also be altered. In additional complication, an impacted amygdala can trigger the release of hormones and chemicals in the body.

When the amount of cortisol as well as other elements in brain chemistry is balanced, shrinkage of the hippocampus occurs. Achieving this balance can address memory problems and reduce the symptoms of depression.

To do this, medication is a common treatment. Several prescription medications are successful in balancing brain chemistry. Some of the most commonly prescribed are:

- Selective Serotonin Uptake Inhibitors (SSRI)
- Serotonin-Norepinephrine Reuptake Inhibitors (SNRI) and Tricyclic Antidepressants:
- Norepinephrine-Dopamine Reuptake Inhibitors (NDRIs)
- Monoamine Oxidase Inhibitors (MAOI)

Serotonin, norepinephrine, and dopamine improve both energy and mood levels, as well as act on brain cell communication. The following pharmaceutical classification allows the body to relax, thus suppressing brain cell communication and slowing down the production and release of cortisol.

- Atypical Antidepressants: Included in this group are mood stabilizers, tranquilizers, and antipsychotics.

Therapy is also an option in helping to restore brain function. Some examples of the therapy often used to correct the brain chemistry imbalances are:

- Electroconvulsive therapy (ECT) – to improve brain cell communication, electrical current is passed through the brain.
- Transcranial magnetic stimulation (TMS) – targets the brain's ability to regulate mood by directing electric pulses into the cells of the brain charged with this function.

The third method of that has shown some success in research is psychotherapy. The definition of psychotherapy is simply therapy which occurs between an individual and a trained mental health therapist in which psychological issues are examined. It is believed that therapy sessions like this relieve depression symptoms and help change the way in which the prefrontal cortex part of the brain responds.

In addition, doctors often recommend that a person suffering from depression can also make healthy choices, especially those that directly impact brain health. These healthy choices include eating nutritional foods and pursuing an active lifestyle, both of which boost brain cell communication. Getting plenty of sleep is found to grow brain cells as well as repair damaged cells.

Suicide – Myths of Suicide

About 41,000 people committed suicide in a single year. An estimated 1.3 million adults have attempted suicide, and 2.7 adults have voiced the intention to commit suicide. Mental health researchers estimate that 9.3 million adults have suicidal thought.

Statistics indicate that women are more likely to attempt suicide, but men are more likely to die from suicide.

Suicidal thoughts are a serious consequence of depression. About half of those who attempt suicide have been diagnosed with a mental health disorder. What prevents many people from seeking help are some of the misinformation that surrounds suicide and suicidal thoughts.

For the rest of those who attempt or commit suicide, the self-destructive tendency is prompted by a number of stress factors occurring in a person's life. These could be related to relationships, trouble with the law, financial problems, death of someone close, trauma, abuse, dealing with a devastating illness and other situations which cause high levels of stress and are deeply emotional to the person.

As with many other health conditions, there are some risk factors for suicide. These include: someone who has attempted suicide in the past; someone who has experienced a stressful life event; someone with a substance abuse problem; someone who has a mental health disorder; has mental health issues that run in the family; someone who has a medical condition linked to depression; and someone who is lesbian, gay, bisexual or transgender without family support.

Suicide can be prevented. Intervention by someone if a person is showing any of the warning signs can literally save a life.

If anyone is considering suicide, reach out for help. Speak to a family member or close friend. Contact a member of the faith community to talk about your feelings and thoughts. Make an appointment with your doctor.

Call 911 or a local emergency number. Call a hotline to speak with someone who can help. The National Suicide Prevention Lifeline is 1-800-273 TALK. Veterans can also call that number and press "1."

- **Myth: A suicidal person will always be suicidal.**

Research indicates that suicidal intentions are short-term and are usually situation-specific. With proper treatment, these thoughts and intentions can be controlled.

People consider suicide when they are dealing with powerful emotions and deeply wounding thoughts that are not being controlled. If the thoughts are managed and lose their intensity, the idea of committing suicide goes away.

- Myth: Most suicides happen without warning.

Individuals who are entertaining thoughts of suicide often exhibit warning signs, either verbally or in the way that person is behaving. Sometimes these warning signs are observed by those the person feels closest too. Outside of family and friends, these thoughts, and behaviors are kept secret.

Although warning signs don't come highlighted or with a flashing light to draw someone's attention, there are signals that often point to a person's suicidal state of mind. Warning signs of suicide include:

- ✓ Avoiding and withdrawing from contact with family and friends and expressing the desire to be left alone
- ✓ Extreme mood swings, from very happy and optimistic to very sad and pessimistic, in a matter of hours
- ✓ Talking about killing themselves or expressing, "I wish I were dead," or similar comments.
- ✓ A preoccupation with violence, death and dying
- ✓ Increased substance abuse
- ✓ Increased risky or dangerous behavior
- ✓ A change in sleeping or eating patterns
- ✓ Taking steps to acquire the means to end a life
- ✓ Giving away belongings or putting affairs in order when there appears to be no reason

- ✓ Expressing a feeling of being trapped or hopeless in a situation

- Myth: Suicide is a result of depression.

When the numbers of people who are diagnosed with depression are compared with the number of people who commit suicide, it becomes obvious that this myth is untrue. Many people who are clinically depressed do not attempt or commit suicide.

It is estimated that about half of those who die from suicide were also depressed and may also have had other psychological disorders.

While suicide is a consequence of depression, it is not the only consequence.

- Myth: Suicides are not something that can be stopped.

Evidence suggests that prevention efforts make a difference and results in the savings of countless lives every day. People who are suicidal or those who talk about suicide are sending out signals about the seriousness of their mental state. These signals are some of the warning signs that others need to cue in on.

When these warning signs are heeded, it is possible to stop someone from taking their life. Early indications that symptoms are compounding should be the call for action.

Suicide often happens as a response to the difficulties adding up.

- Myth: Talking about suicide encourages suicide.

Suicide is seldom talked about because it carries a stigma, but this topic needs to be given a voice. When suicide is discussed, it lessens the stigma and provides a way for people to seek help.

Especially when suicide is discussed on a clinical level, people who may be contemplating suicide are provided with options, facts, and resources to allow them to seek the help they need. Talking about suicide doesn't encourage it; it prevents it.

- Myth: Suicide doesn't happen to young children.

Each year about 30 children in the United States under the age of 12 commit suicide. The research on this occurrence is still incomplete, but it does happen. Prevention efforts are not typically targeting this age group.

- Myth: The act of suicide is an impulsive one.

Suicide is actually most often a planned act. The person who is considering suicide will have given it much thought, hinted at their intentions, and planned out the act, perhaps even writing final letters to loved ones. It may take as short as several days to a few weeks to reach the point in which a suicide occurs.

Suicides among children, however, are more impulsive, but there will still be signs. Perhaps the child has told a friend, discussed suicide in school work or dropped hints to an adult at school.

- Myth: Suicide is an easy way out.

According to mental health experts, people are wrong to think that suicide is all about ending life. It is a solution to ending a person's pain. The feeling of hopelessness caused by the mental anguish and the deeply emotional state the person is under is the motivation for considering suicide. People who are suicidal also feel helpless in finding a solution to relieve their emotional state.

These individuals are in a troubled mental health state. Their decision making is compromised because of the huge emotional burden they carry.

The best way to dispel the myths about suicide is to talk about it. Confronting falsehoods about this mental health issue is the best way to make sure that those who need help are poised to receive it.

What Happens When Depression Gets Serious?

There is no doubt that suicide is a serious consequence of depression. There are treatment options that can help. Clinical depression that does not get treated has serious consequences. It increases the probability of substance abuse and drug addiction, can interfere with relationships and the ability to work.

It also puts the physical body at risk. Evidence suggests that depression can impede a heart attack or stroke survivors' ability to make health care decisions, follow treatment protocol and coping with the challenges of recovery. A study also found that a heart patient with depression has a more likely chance of dying within the first few months after suffering a heart attack.

Untreated depression also manifests strongly in men. In these cases, men tend to demonstrate more rage and frustration. They may become more violent with women. They often take risks that are dangerous, such as unsafe sex, driving recklessly and other potentially life-threatening actions.

Depression is considered a disability because it seriously affects the way people live their lives. Job performance, family life and even social interactions with friends are impacted when someone is in a depressed state. Statistics indicate that sick days lost from work because of untreated depression cost more than $43 billion in costs, with 200 million-plus days of work lost.

When dealing with a family member who has depression, especially a child or teen, the parent should offer support on an emotional level. Patience, encouragement, and understanding are key to helping a family member cope with the emotional toll of depression.

Conversations should be meaningful, and not necessarily about depression. Listen carefully to what the family member or friend is saying. It is important to offer a perspective on reality as well as hope without disregarding the depressed person's feelings. Remind them that depression will prolong life, with treatment and as time goes on.

Some comments require immediate attention, like those that express a desire to hurt themselves or others and those that reference suicide.

Addiction is another possible outcome when depression is untreated. Ignoring the symptoms of depression is not a treatment option. Lack of a treatment plan to combat the symptoms of depression often leaves those exhibiting the symptoms to turn to self-medicating with drugs or alcohol. Besides the risk of developing an addiction, drugs and alcohol can make the symptoms even more pronounced.

Self-harm is another example of how untreated depression can develop into a serious consequence. Although the intention of self-harm is not to severely injure or cause death, cutting and burning can go wrong. Accidents happen, and death can occur.

Taking chances that are dangerous or reckless are also more likely to happen if the symptoms of depression are not addressed. Feelings of low self-worth, hopelessness, and anger often influence depressed people to make poor choices.

Chapter 5: Managing Depression

Depression is a serious condition that requires treatment to alleviate the symptoms and keep the disorder from becoming more serious. In addition to medical and therapeutic intervention, there are numerous ways to keep the symptoms of depression from impacting your life more than necessary.

Any illness or affliction can be helped with some non-clinical methods—such as finding the right combination of diet, sleep, and physical activity that improve brain and body function, balance psychological and physiological imbalances, and help repair damaged cells.

Like any type of management program, a planned approach is necessary, and a commitment to work the program as needed is essential. Especially when dealing with a disorder that can impact daily life and social interactions, developing a routine of positive actions can make a difference.

Many of the ways to manage depression are beneficial in reducing stress. Stressful situations stimulate the body to release higher levels of cortisol and other hormones needed in response to the body's defensive mechanisms. Controlling the levels of stress as much as possible will lead to an overall improved brain chemistry balance.

Boost Your Self-Esteem

People struggling with depression or other disorders like social anxiety have been found to have low self-esteem, self-confidence, and a heightened sense of self-consciousness. Improving self-esteem is an all-around good idea. Research has shown that people who have confidence and a high regard for their sense of self tend to be healthier and more successful.

This is a critical world. The immediate gratification found in social media means that people don't often censor themselves when it comes to leaving negative reviews or even when insults are directed at others. No one likes to be insulted or criticized—but in the end, the most important opinion is the one we have of ourselves. And sometimes, a person is harder on themselves than on another person.

Self-esteem building is a difficult task—mostly because a person has to learn to silence the internal critic and avoid comparing themselves to others. For someone who is already experiencing anxiety about what others think about them, the inner voice that feeds these fears is the enemy. Luckily, there are experts who have come up with some ways to allow a person to take control and work on improving their self-esteem.

Gaining the ability to recognize negative thoughts as simply a thought and not irrefutable proof of inabilities is a key element in being mindful. Trying to ignore the judgmental inner voice does not adequately address the situation. Being aware of how the thoughts affect the self-esteem, recognizing that these thoughts are not facts, and learning when the rationale is needed to confront the negative and substitute the positive.

What a person believes is true about their life becomes the narrative they recite and forms the judgments they make about themselves. If that narrative is one-sided, it dictates the direction of self-esteem. A positive narrative automatically raises the person's self-worth, while a negative storyline allows negative thoughts to have the most influence. To change this dynamic, a person needs to change the story.

Experts say that a person learns to communicate the negative thoughts about themselves and that replacing these with positive ones can change the inner conversation. What was once learned can be unlearned, or at least that knowledge can be replaced with a better and positive affirmation.

Affirmations are a way to replace the negative viewpoint with one that reflects the truth about ourselves. One way to zero in on the best qualities and skills is for an individual to make a list of the positive elements in his or her life, especially those that he or she possesses. Giving this a time limit forces the brain to focus on qualities that represent the positive.

In addition to the list providing information to begin changing self-criticism, it also serves as a tool for reducing the effect of some symptoms of depression.

Rekindling interest in what makes a person happy is a way to invigorate a person's self-esteem. Identifying the activities or skills a person does well is a balance to the things that they do not do well. For example, some people are great at fixing things, such as computers, but they may not be able to sing. Someone may be a fantastic photographer but can't play tennis. It is important to remember that no one does everything well. Everyone has strengths and weaknesses.

Volunteering or engaging in charitable work is also a way to rev up self-esteem. When a person devotes time and energy to help others, the focus is no longer on themselves, but on the difference, their efforts are making in other people's lives.

Lending a hand to help those less fortunate generates a good feeling, one that affirms the goodness within.

The pay-it-forward initiative is an example of how one kind act can have a ripple effect on others. When a person does something nice for another person, it creates a sense of satisfaction and accomplishment, generating a positive response in the emotion center of the brain.

Don't underestimate the power of forgiveness. Learning to forgive and let go is a way to discard the negative memories that weigh down a person's mood. Research suggests that granting forgiveness to those who been hurtful affects self-esteem. Doing so allows us to accept the shortcomings of others, generates a more loving nature and provides closure needed to move on.

The Healthy Brain (SEEDS)

There is evidence that maintaining a healthy brain can provide a way to keep depression and other anxiety disorders from becoming too severe. In terms of increasing brain health and improving cognitive awareness and function, taking an all-encompassing approach to whole body health has been a successful program for people suffering from age-related degenerative diseases, such as Alzheimer's disease.

According to research, a focus on maintaining a healthy mind improves the body's health as well and lessens the possibility of developing cognitive problems later in life. A program with the acronym SEEDS has been used with Alzheimer patients. SEEDS is Sleep, Eat, Exercise, Domain, and Social Engagement.

Individually, any of these five components are healthy for the mind and body.

Sleep gives the brain time to cleanse itself of toxins.

Healthy food choices and intermittent fasting keep the body's metabolic functions functioning well, providing nutrients to the organs and the brain.

Physical activity keeps muscles and joints fluid and releases hormones that contribute to brain and body health.

Maintaining a toxin-free living space reduces contamination and limits exposure to toxins that may be detrimental to the brain and body.

And finally, being socially active helps boost spirits and elevate mood.

Socialization

One of the symptoms of depression is a withdrawal from social situations. Sometimes depression results in isolation from friends, family, and people in general. The opportunities to interact with others become limited by depression, especially when the disorder keeps a person from going to work, attending school or visiting with other people. Interacting with others can be stressful, but it makes sense that adding a socializing element to depression management works.
People who are struggling with depression often avoid contact with people they know and people to whom they are close. They avoid doing things that were once enjoyed with others. As it worsens, people will avoid any contact with other people, including not answering the phone or returning phone calls.

Much of this avoidance comes out of fear that friends or family will judge them or that the symptoms of depression may be too much to handle for those who know and love you. The thought of meeting new people when a person is overwhelmed with debilitating emotions is not a consideration.

To keep depression from getting to the point where a person becomes isolated, making an effort to mingle with others, have a conversation, or experience a shared interest is an effective way to minimize the progression of symptoms. Studies indicate that people who socialize are less likely to become depressed and those who distance themselves from social contact are at risk of becoming depressed.

People who have been diagnosed with depression or social anxiety feel alone in their struggle. That feeling is compounded by the lack of contact with others. Being alone feels unnatural to the human psyche, based on the communal lifestyle of the human experience.

Besides lessening loneliness, socialization draws a person out of their focus on their problems and worries. Sharing the experience of dinner out, a movie, a walk in the park, a visit to an art gallery, or any other activity changes perspective from inward to outward. It is a break from the confines of depression.

But socialization does not have to involve going somewhere or doing something unless the person is ready for that type of interaction. A phone call or online chat with a friend is a terrify mood booster. Slipping away for a coffee break with a coworker is another way to make socialization fit into a daily routine.

Taking a step toward building new friendships can also be part of the socialization component of depression management. It may not be a strategy someone may want to try early in the treatment process but can be helpful as the depression symptoms lighten or to maintain a depression-free state of mind.

Think about getting in touch with people with whom you may have lost contact. A friend who stood by you in the tough times and enjoyed better times is someone that can be added back into your life. There's a familiarity that takes away the nervousness that comes from meeting someone new.

Expanding your existing circle of friends is also a way to use socialization as a strategy for managing depression. There are many opportunities to meet new people by volunteering at organizations for which you have a passion. If you are an animal lover, the humane society could be a place to volunteer which puts you in contact with like-minded individuals. Your place of worship can also open up new acquaintances as well as adding to the availability of people to support you in a spiritual sense.

Enrolling in a class at a college or university in the community also increases the opportunities to socialize. Sign up for an art class, a dance class, or take golf or tennis lessons. Chances are there will be people there who share the same interest.

Getting out in the community and being around people is a positive approach to controlling the symptoms of depression. It may take some effort to take the first steps, to reach out a hand in friendship, to get past the nervousness of first-time introductions. Friends add value to life and give us a companion to take on a journey.

Education

When someone has not been diagnosed with depression, the symptoms can be scary. You don't understand why you feel the way you do and why you have lost the pleasure in life. This confusion comes from not knowing what is causing the symptoms you are experiencing.

But when you have been diagnosed, there are opportunities to learn more about depression. You suddenly know what to search for in looking for information about the disorder and what you can do to make life better.

When a person is armed with information and knowledge, this is a powerful tool to use in fighting the consequences that come with the disorder. Seeking information to understand what is happening when a person is depressed is a way to manage the progression and remission of depression.

Becoming knowledgeable about depression is important for the person with depression as well as caregivers. Knowing the symptoms of depression, treatment options and resources available improve shed light on a subject for which a person may not have needed to know prior to the diagnosis.

Learning about depression also exposes the person to the stories of others who have faced similar challenges. Finding similarities and differences in these personal accounts helps to highlight the understanding that depression is much more common than people think.

Taking control of your own care and treatment options is empowering. Having a solid understanding of depression also creates teachable moments. Conversations about depression can now be supported with the knowledge acquired as part of the management strategy.

Exercise

Being active, at whatever level a person is capable of being, has long been a way to not only maintain a healthy body but a way to boost energy, mood, and balance brain and body chemistry. Regular exercise has a positive influence on self-esteem as well as reducing stress.

Research has indicated that exercise strengthens the body, improves the body's ability to metabolize food, and generates a general feeling of accomplishment. It is a route to better self-care because the attention has to be focused on the individual and not what is going on around them.

Effective exercise requires an activity that forces the heart rate to rise in response. This increases blood flow to the brain and the body. Better blood flow means the body's most vital organs are getting what they need to function properly. Studies have shown there is a correlation between physical activity and a reduced risk of cognitive function.

Exercise doesn't have to resemble an athlete training for the Olympics. Instead, it is recommended that each person finds the activity and activity level that is comfortable but effective for their personal needs. Gym memberships are one option, but so is going on a walk with a friend, joining a dance class, gardening, or taking the dog for a walk. Making exercise an enjoyable experience ensures that the person will continue to do it on a regular basis.

Choosing to park farther away from the door allows a few extra steps into a person's daily count. Opting to walk up a flight of stairs is also an effective way of adding more activity into the routine.

The connection between exercise and the brain is well documented. Being physically active stimulates the growth of new nerve cells and improves the response of synapses, the connections between the brain's cells.

Diet

A newly emerging field of psychology suggests that diet has more effect on brain function and psychological disorders than previously thought. Dubbed Nutritional Psychiatry, the idea is that a proper diet is the best way to ensure that the brain stays healthy and that the body has what it needs to circumvent adverse reactions to stressful situations.

Fuel for the brain is supplied by a person's diet. Just like the fuel put into car engines, the higher the grade, the better the performance. For the human body, however, it is all about providing the healthiest combination of foods in the right quantity. The best foods are high in vitamins, minerals, and antioxidants. These high-octane foods are free from preservatives and chemicals used in processing.

Processed foods with high sugar content are detrimental to the body because it directly affects the body's control of insulin. It also promotes inflammation and can contribute to oxidation stress. Research has noted a high sugar diet's effect on the brain as well. It has been shown that this type of diet messes with brain function and can compound the symptoms of depression and mood disorders.

Eating the proper foods ensures that all physiological functions operate properly and that all the systems release the hormones and neurotransmitters needed to keep brain chemistry balanced. As an example, consider that serotonin normalizes appetite and sleep. Serotonin is produced in the gastrointestinal tract, which is also responsible for digesting food. In addition, the bacteria in the digestive system help cleanse the body of toxins.

Research has shown that these good bacteria – probiotics – are essential to the digestive system and regulate the connections between the nerve cells and the brain. When these are at a high level, anxiety, and stress decreases and overall mental health improves.

The choice of foods can also influence brain health and reduce the risk of depression or other disorders. Opting for a so-called traditional diet, like those consumed in the Mediterranean or Japanese cultures, can reduce the risk of depression by up to 35 percent, according to research. Fruits and vegetables, and unprocessed grains are plentiful in traditional diets. So too are fish and seafood. Missing from these diets are processed foods and refined sugars.

Sleep

The obvious reason to include a healthy sleep cycle as part of a program to managing depression is that it provides the rest that the body and mind needs. Sleep also removes toxins from the brain. The buildup of these toxins happens while the person is awake and moving through the course of the day. This important brain cleansing activity is important to research when looking at the connection between a lack of sleep and depression.

When someone is not sleeping well, health experts know that there is an effect on the brain and body. Sleep deficiency weakens the ability to solve problems, notice details, and mars the power to reason.

When someone is tired, they are less productive in their jobs. Their attention is compromised, putting them at risk for an accident. Lack of sleep makes a person irritable, making interactions with others terse. Lack of sleep for an extended period is a risk factor for developing depression.

Lack of sleep can also raise the risk of getting seriously ill. It raises the risk of a person being diagnosed with heart disease and infections.

Recent research has shown that the brain's cleansing action removes a protein called a beta-amyloid, which has been detected in high quantities in the brains of Alzheimer patients. This research matches findings that suggest that the levels of beta-amyloid decrease while a person is asleep.

While a person sleeps, their body is still working. Heart rate, blood pressure, and breathing rate fluctuate throughout the night as the body balances the system. Hormones produced and circulated while the person is asleep repair cells and regulate energy use and absorption.

To keep the body and brain functioning well, experts recommend between 7 – 9 hours of sleep for adults. Teenagers function better on nine hours of sleep, children should get at least 10 hours, and infants sleep for 16 hours.

Minimizing the distractions are one way to make sure a person slips easily into sleep. The light from electronic devices is especially distracting. Drinking coffee or other caffeine-rich beverages before sleep can impact a person's ability to fall asleep. Some medications have a similar effect.

Use of Self-Love and Self-Compassion

Self-love is difficult for people who are struggling with depression. In many cases, a person's self-worth and connections to others are fractured, and even the simplest task takes tremendous effort. Putting a priority on yourself is not on the list when simply getting through the day is the challenge.

Self-Love is treating yourself with care. It's taking care of your needs so you are better able to focus on maintaining your depression or anxiety disorder. It doesn't involve lots of money or effort, just seeing that personal needs are attended to.

First, eat foods that are good for your body and your brain. You might think that a candy bar and potato chips may fill that void, but a healthy breakfast, lunch, and dinner with plenty of vegetables, fruits, whole grains, and proteins are a better choice. Make sure that the calories you provide your body are the kind that will be converted to energy and supply the vitamins and minerals your brain and body need.

Proper nutrition does not have to be complicated, especially when depression makes you not want to do much of anything. Make an effort to choose healthier quick and easy meal options/

Second, take care of your hygiene. Taking a shower, washing our hair and doing other tasks related to cleanliness is difficult for those with depression. Even a quick washing up, the use of a dry shampoo and brushing your teeth is a start. Try to do more than the bare minimum in the hygiene department, such as taking a shower or bath. A bath is particularly soothing and healing.

Soak up the Vitamin D. Get outside. Go for a walk. Sit in a park. Watch the ducks at the lake. These simple and low energy activities are great for enhancing mood. There are calmness and peaceful feelings that come from being outside. Carving out a little time during the day or evening to venture outside is good for you and shows you care about your mind, body, and spirit.

Rediscover your pleasure. Do you remember what made you happy? Was it art or poetry? Knitting or woodworking? Tinkering with your motorcycle or reading a book? Maybe it is watching made-for-television movies or relaxing to your favorite musical artist. Taking time to do things that you like to do is a great way to show yourself some love.

In a state of depression, indulging in this kind of activities may seem impossible. Simply try. Don't pressure yourself into finishing that masterpiece or the Great American Novel. Start small and enjoy the moment.

The second part of this depression management equation is self-compassion. This term means to find the dignity and wisdom in your experience and respond with kindness. Put aside the common depression-related thought that there is something wrong with you; that the world is too dark of a place; or that you have no purpose in this life. None of this is true and finding a way to show yourself some compassion will help lessen the impact of these feelings.

Touch is one way to be compassionate. One suggestion is to place your hand on your heart and take a deep breath. Or, simply brush your hand against your face or your arm. Touch stimulates the receptors in the skin, triggering a feeling of compassion.

Delve into your experiences. Writing down observations in a journal or expressing your feelings in a sketchbook. Making a connection with your own depression or negative thoughts is the same as talking with a friend and getting or giving advice.

Taking action to find solutions to your depression is also therapeutic and shows compassion. It demonstrates that you are making an effort to get better and that you are taking the steps to reclaim your power.

Practice Mindfulness – Be in the Moment

Mindfulness meditation is a way to focus on the present and not the past, in which the incidents, people or situations occurred that affected your brain and body's ability to move beyond stress and anxiety. Being in the present means taking stock of what is going on within and around your body and brain. When being mindful, the awareness of where we are, what we are doing is highlighted.

Over time, human beings who are depressed or diagnosed with an anxiety disorder have become accustomed to zeroing in on the negative aspects of life experiences. People remember when they were embarrassed, made a mistake, humiliated in front of others, or faced some other situation which allowed a criticism of themselves to be lodged in their memory. These emotionally devastating moments have become the way in which a person views themselves but are just some of the life experiences that contribute to who a person is.

Mindfulness helps by shifting focus from bad experiences to positive ones. It takes away the process of judging feelings and emotions and substitutes a more analytical and observational quality to a person's perceptions of themselves.

By eliminating the need to reflect on the past or worry about the future, mindfulness helps dissipate negative thoughts by assigning neither a positive or negative label on these. It is simply living in the present, experiencing what it is like to live in the now.

Personal perceptions of time are not simply objective observations but carry emotions as well. These memories of the past and worries about the future are linked to fears and anxiety. That makes it problematic to give these perceptions their deserved importance. Through mindfulness, enjoyment comes from the present.

Being mindful is focusing on what is happening with our bodies, our minds, and our emotions. The techniques of mindfulness are simple and do not require anyone to adopt a new belief system. It works within the structure of what a person already believes and knows about themselves.

Mindfulness forces the body to relax through focused concentration. It asks the person to be aware of their breathing, how their body curves and bends, how their heartbeat feels and sounds.

The benefit of mindfulness in the scope of managing depression is that the practice of it can naturally encourage the body to relax. When the body relaxes, the natural rhythms of the body calm the nerves and slows any signs of agitation. Less stress means the body and brain function better and the person's health, in general, improves.

Knowing how to do this gives a person with depression a tool to use when needed. Because mindfulness requires no fancy equipment or a specific place to go, it can easily be used to calm nerves or get passed a tough time of the day.

The ritual begins with deep, slow and rhythmic breaths. The eyes close and the practitioner moves through the parts of the body calling for a focus followed by relaxation. As the practitioner continues, the goal is to achieve a relaxed state from head to toe.

Mindfulness exercises are not complex and do not require an enormous amount of effort. Simple exercises can be used to achieve mindfulness meditation easily.

One technique is simply to observe the events and happening going on around you. The world moves at a very fast pace. While practicing mindfulness that pace slows down. Paying attention to how the body's five senses are responding while eating, visiting a park, or petting a dog is a mindfulness exercise that can be practiced anytime and anyplace.

A second method is to make an effort to focus on everything the practitioner does. In other words, live right now. Pamper yourself, celebrate the unpretentious joys in life, practice self-acceptance. Counter negative thoughts by focusing on deep, slow breathing to let the negative thoughts fade away.

Another exercise that mixes physical activity with mindfulness is walking meditation. According to instructions, the person should seek out a quiet place that allows about 10 – 20 feet of walking space. The person then begins to walk slowly across space. The mindfulness experience focuses on the act of walking, taking in the movements the body makes and how a person balances as the activity is underway. At the end of the path, turn around and continue to walk, constantly practicing being mindful of the experience as well as how the body responds.

Mindfulness exercises fit neatly into the sometimes-hectic schedules of everyday life. Although these meditations can be done anywhere, there is an added benefit if the mindfulness meditation is conducted outside. The suggested duration for this depression management technique is at least six months.

For more structured mindfulness exercises, such as body scan meditation or sitting meditation, you'll need to set aside time when you can be in a quiet place without distractions or interruptions. You might choose to practice this type of exercise early in the morning before you begin your daily routine.

Aim to practice mindfulness every day for about six months. Over time, you might find that mindfulness becomes effortless. Think of it as a commitment to reconnecting with and nurturing yourself.

Chapter 6: Wrapping It Up – Strategies and Resources

Depression, anxiety disorders, and phobias are not like medical illnesses—many of which there are no cures. Instead, someone who is suffering from depression or has social anxiety can take an active role in making themselves feel better.

A healthy diet, exercise, meditation, and other techniques can enhance any clinical treatments or medical interventions. While it is not wise to go through it alone without the help of a mental health professional, managing depression is a proactive and self-compassionate act.

Check Your Progression on Overcoming Social Anxiety or Depression

As with any goal a person sets for themselves, if an individual is taking steps to help themselves manage depression, it is important to know how to measure progress. Keep in mind that there will be ups and downs on the journey, but the most important consideration is to keep trying.

The easiest way to track progress is to set up a journal or record to assess what is going on. There are online resources that provide direct questions that can help track improvements and provide an objective measurement instead of a subjective one. Finding out what progress has been made is as simple as asking questions and recording the responses.

When you are training your body in preparation for an athletic event, there are measurements that can be taken to assess conditioning, tone, weight gain or loss, and heart rate among other tools to objectively measure the progress that has been made. There are no measurements that can be taken to determine if the methods being used to manage depression and anxiety are working. A person cannot simply look in the mirror and see a difference in their brain. It is important that a person listens to their thoughts to determine if their inner dialogue has changed.

Be prepared to ask yourself some tough questions and commit to answering as honestly as you can. Don't simply accept the automatic answer your mind suggests—review it and decide if it is an accurate reflection of your efforts.

Is your day-to-day functioning showing improvement? To determine if there are signs of improvement, set short-term goals, such as committing to missing fewer days of work or school or getting more sleep. As you achieve these initial short-term goals, set new ones.

Do you see an improvement with your symptoms? The Wakefield Questionnaire is a tool to rate your answers to specific questions to calculate a numeric score. This score can be compared along the way to any changes.

When completing the Wakefield Questionnaire, participants are asked to indicate on a scale of zero to three their response to the statement. One of the first questions on this form is to respond to the question I feel miserable and sad. The response includes: No, not at all (0), No, not much (1), Yes, sometimes (2), and Yes, definitely (3). Other questions include whether the person finds it easy to do the things he or she used to do, if they feel panicked or frightened for no reason, and if he or she has weeping spells or feels like crying. A similar questionnaire may have been given to the person when first consulting a medical or mental health professional.

By adding up the number value for each response, the total can determine the severity of the depression. A score above 15, indicates a person is likely depressed. Tests like the Wakefield Questionnaire are not intended to be used to diagnose clinical depression. It is a tool or gauges the possibility that a person may be depressed.

By repeating the Wakefield Questionnaire as a person continues treatment is a way to see if there has been an improvement. Although the responses are subjective to the individual, it can be useful to identify changes in responses.

Another self-test for depression takes a little different approach to the questions. The Zung Self-Rating Depression Scale asks the person to rate 20 statements on their physical and emotional state based on a scale of A little of the time, Some of the time, A good part of the time and Most of the time. Each response has a point value. Respondents are asked to answer statements such as I feel downhearted and blue; I feel I am useful and needed, and My mind is as clear as it used to be.

Examples of these and other assessments are available from multiple online sources. If using one of these tests to determine progress, make sure the same one is used each time. Different tests have different scoring systems, and that could affect the interpretation of progress in the treatment program.

Have there been any relapses? If your depression symptoms are under control, that indicates improvement. Managing depression is important because the chances of someone with depression having another occurrence of depression is increased.

Have lifestyle changes been made successfully? Changing the habits of daily life can help improve depression, especially if the situations or events that are considered stressors are under control. These lifestyle changes include being healthy and active, relating to others in a more inclusive and positive way, and dealing with stress in a proactive manner.

Lastly, consider whether your medications are causing side effects or are effective in your treatment. Treatments such as prescription drugs are designed to address some of the physiological symptoms of depression, such as stabilizing brain chemistry. If the medication side effects are complicating your life or impacting your abilities to manage your depression, your medical or mental health provider needs to know. Frustration with difficult side effects can lead to discouragement and short-circuit your progress.

There are also applications that can be downloaded on devices that are engineered to help with depression. These apps serve multiple purposes, from providing information on depression to providing tools for self-assessment. Other apps monitor physiological processes, such as heart rate, the rate of breathing and pulse. Others also have a way to determine the stress level.

To make the best choice in an app, find one that works for you that is science-based if that is what you need. Look for information on how the app obtains its information, such as from a consultation with medical or mental health experts.

There are a variety of apps that focus on the various treatment options, such as one that addresses cognitive behavior therapy. An app dealing with this treatment option provides information on the therapy and has a test to help a person determine the severity of the depression. This is an electronic version of the paper versions of the various depression questionnaires. As a tool to measure progress, the app has a tracking component to record positive thoughts and overall mood. It also includes guided meditations for those with depression.

One app that has received an endorsement from mental health professionals who were also designers of the program is called MoodKit. This app is designed to help someone overcome a bad mood by providing mood improvement activities. There are other apps that provide similar support. The journal tool and built-in thought tracker on MoodKit and other apps provide a resource for recording thoughts or observations. Its primary function is to elevate the mood of the user.

Other apps, such as Daylio, allows the user to record their mood, using an emoji-like system. Tools built into apps like this provide a visual record of the emotional swings. Like many of these self-assessment apps, there is usually a journaling feature.

Remember that an app is not a replacement for professional mental health advice. Consult with your doctor before following any suggestions made by an online or mobile source.

Talk to Someone

Anyone who is experiencing any of the symptoms of depression or an anxiety disorder should remember that they do not have to go it alone. In fact, being able to talk about the diagnosis or the challenges is both therapeutic and essential in getting the help a person needs in managing depression.

Reaching out to family and friends is a convenient way to begin the conversation about your mental health. These are often the people you trust the most, the ones whom you know have your back when things get tough. Consider the family members who have the personality to be the most supportive. Someone who is judgmental or pessimistic may not be the person to whom you open up to.

Finding the words to express how depression or anxiety is impacting your life is not an easy task. There is no set of instructions to follow to convey what you feel, what you experience or what obstacles you scale every day. Remember that everyone is an expert on themselves and depression is different for everyone.

If family and friends are an uncomfortable option to begin a conversation about your mental health challenges, seek out another person you trust. A teacher is one option; a member of the clergy can be another. Perhaps there is a counselor or medical professional you have a rapport with that could be someone to listen as you vocalize what you are feeling inside.

Bringing another person or persons into the loop is a good first step toward finding a way out. Giving your inner thoughts a voice can be therapeutic.

Don't be afraid to ask for help and support. Developing a strong support network and making use of their love and commitment to your health is vital and an important treatment tool.

Aside from family and friends, one important person to include in these conversations about depression is the primary care doctor. The symptoms of depression are similar to symptoms for other health concerns. A primary care doctor can narrow down the diagnoses to make sure the problems the patient is experiencing is related to depression.

When you need to find a new doctor for any reason, take some time to find a practitioner that can relate to you and with whom you are comfortable. You will be sharing some very personal information, and the ability to trust the medical professional is important.

A medical doctor may be only the first step in finding your way to treatment and relief from depression. You may be referred to a mental health professional for further evaluation. Be prepared to talk about family history of depression or other mental illness, as well as the list of your symptoms.

Finding a support group is a good option in finding people to talk to about depression. The experience of sharing information, feelings, strategies, and tips about treatments and managing depression from those who are living with it like you are is encouraging and helpful.

Talk to your support group about the challenges you face and the treatment plan that has been put in place by your mental health team. Talk about what triggers anxiety or stress and seek their support in helping you make better lifestyle choices.

While some support groups meet in person, there are other options for someone who would be more comfortable participating in an online chat room for people with depression. It is important to look for a chat room moderated or affiliated with a mental health organization. The online chat room also provides more anonymity in conversations while providing a community of people who can identify with a person's struggles with depression.

Chat rooms that are moderated are a safe place to share experiences. Open social media platforms are not. It is important to remember that very few of the chat rooms will have a mental health professional as the moderator. While most do their best to maintain a safe, polite environment, there is no guarantee that discussions may not turn hostile. Chat rooms should be used as an additional resource in addition to seeking help from professionals in the mental health or medical community.

Talk therapy is one of the treatment options available in the fight against depression. Also known as psychotherapy, it involves a client and a therapist. The therapy session usually lasts no more than an hour and can take different directions, depending on the treatment plan or any current crises in a person's life that require attention.

There are several types of psychotherapy. Variations include cognitive-behavioral, interpersonal and problem-solving therapies.

Access to a therapist in a digital world is a possibility. Research indicates that many people achieve positive results with online therapy programs, but mental health practitioners caution people from going this route without checking credentials and clearing the treatment program with your doctor.

When someone is talking to you about their depression, there is no script to follow. The best way to respond is to listen to what they say and show them you support them. Assuring them that you are ready to help in any way you can or reminding them that they do not have to handle this alone are positive ways to respond.

It's also acceptable to ask someone if they are OK, even if the inquiry seems awkward or is uncomfortable. It opens a door that a person suffering from depression needs to walk through. Avoid saying that you know how they feel. Don't discount what they are experiencing by saying, "everyone gets depressed" or "think happy thoughts." And don't tell them they have nothing to be depressed about.

What happens when a person's mental health has reached a crisis stage, such as the contemplation of suicide? At this life-or-death moment, it is even more important for the person contemplating taking this step to reach and talk about their feelings. If that person is reluctant to tell family, friends or their support group, there are still people who can help.

The National Suicide Prevention Crisis Center maintains a toll-free hotline to provide that extra help at what could be the darkest moment of someone's depression. These crisis centers are located in communities and are often part of the county or local behavioral health systems. Most of these centers are structured as non-profit organizations, with both mental health professionals and volunteers available 24-hours a day, seven days a week. These centers do not close for holidays and the services provided are free to those who need it.

When making a call to the hotline, the person in crisis will be directed to someone who can help them almost immediately. There is no travel to a medical center, or the need to make multiple calls to find someone to talk to. The person who answers the call is trained in how to offer help. The person who answers the call listens to the caller, determines the effects the problem is having on the individual and provides support. The caller may also be given resources to help in this situation.

Talking about depression or social anxiety is not easy to do. There are still prejudices against people with mental illnesses, and the subject makes people uncomfortable. Sometimes, however, a little discomfort goes a long way towards healing. People who are struggling with depression feel alone, isolated and as if it was a case of themselves against the world. Talking about depression and how it affects a person brings other people into the struggle. There is safety in numbers, and there is healing too.

Get Your Family and Friends On Board!

When navigating the choppy waters of depression, don't be afraid to build a support group around you of your family and friends. Having people that you trust and those who care about you provides strength and courage to face the challenges each day with depression holds.

A strong support system is an essential part of the recovery process. A support group is a vital part of managing depression, according to research. The positive benefits include improved ways of coping with stressful situations and challenges and provide encouragement to make healthier choices. Support groups also help reduce anxiety and depression.

The size and makeup of the group is a personal decision. Small or large, those who are a part of the support group should be committed to helping their loved one find balance and a way to lift depression. Some people in the group may provide emotional support and others may be better at providing financial support or help in other ways.

Avoid people who may make a situation more stressful. Rule out those who are negative. The best support group members are those with a healthy outlook on life and those who are positive in their thoughts and interactions.

The people who come together in support of a loved one who is diagnosed with depression don't necessarily have to be close friends or family. Neighbors and clergy members are also viable options. Pets can be part of the support a person receives.

When a loved one is diagnosed with depression, it affects those they love. Family and friends can lend their support by making sure their loved one gets medical attention and a diagnosis. A person with depression may need a loved one to come with them to a doctor's appointment. They may also need to be reminded to stick with the treatment plan or may need help finding alternative options.

If you are helping to a family member or friend with their depression, keep your conversations judgment-free and be patient as they work through setbacks and challenges. Be emotionally supportive of their efforts and offer encouragement.

Remember that this is a struggle for your family member or friend, but it will also be difficult for you. A person with depression may need support for an extended period. As a caregiver, take time for yourself and don't neglect your own care.

Here are some other suggestions to make the interaction more positive and effective:

- When talking with your loved one, listen carefully to what they say
- Don't ignore any comment about suicide
- Report any suicide warning signs to their doctor
- Offer hope but don't dismiss how they are feeling
- Be there to help them get to doctor's appointments or other therapy
- Involve your family member in activities, such as going for a walk.
- Reiterate that depression will lift over time with treatment

There are some other ways in which family and friends can demonstrate their support and commitment to their loved one's recovery.

Conduct some research on depression. Understanding the basics of the disorder your loved one is going through is a great way to support them. Once you gain an understanding, it is easier to know how you can help and how to verbally express your commitment to their journey towards healing.

Consider becoming a Mental Health First Aid responder, or at least sign up to take the class. Administered by the National Council for Behavioral Health, this class provides participants with the knowledge to identify risk factors, note warning signs and take action when these signs manifest. In addition, participants learn about treatment options, how to determine if someone is having a mental health crisis, choose interventions to help, and how to connect with resources for the individual.

A Mental Health First Aid responder recognizes the importance of early detection and quick intervention. It helps them identify the patterns and symptoms of several mental health disorders, including anxiety disorders and depression. This information equips the family or friend with fact-based information to better serve as a resource their loved one can count on.

Once you've made the commitment to be there for your family member or friend, make sure you reach out to them regularly. Check on how they are, issue an invitation to hang out or offer to help with errands and daily responsibilities.

Depression and anxiety may be different for everyone, but that doesn't mean the fight with these disorders has to be a solitary one. Bringing family and friends to stand with you makes the journey toward a solution a better one. A helping hand to get you through the day, a hand on the shoulder for support, and a sympathetic ear to get you through an emotional crisis are invaluable.

Talking about depression and anxiety is essential in bringing these inner thoughts to light. Once the negative thoughts are out in the light, it is easier to see the fallacies these thoughts hold. Talk is cheap unless it is to share your struggles and impart knowledge to others. Then talk is priceless.

Organizations and Resources

One of the advantages of the digital world is that information and education is literally at our fingertips. As with anything found on the internet, it is important to check the source's information and determine if the site is credible.

Another cautionary warning is to make sure any suggested therapies for depression or anxiety are approved by your own mental health or medical provider.

The following are some of the national organizations that can educate and provide links to resources for depression and anxiety.

- National Alliance on Mental Illness 1-800-950-NAMI (1-800-950-6264)
- Anxiety and Depression Association of America 1-240-485-1001
- National Institute of Mental Health 1-866-615-6464
- Centers for Disease Control and Prevention Division of Mental Health 1-800-CDC-INFO (1-800-232-4636)
- American Psychological Association 1-800-374-2721
- American Psychiatric Association 1-703-907-7300
- American Foundation for Suicide Prevention 1-800-273-TALK (1-800-273-8255)
- Depression and Bipolar Support Alliance 1-800-826-3632
- Erika's Lighthouse 847-386-6481. This site builds awareness around teenage depression.
- Families for Depression Awareness 1-781-890-0220

Conclusion

Thank you for making it through to the end of Social Anxiety: Guide to Overcome Anxiety and Shyness.

Let's hope it was informative and able to provide you with all of the tools you need to achieve your goals—whatever they may be.

There is a lot of information packed into these six chapters. That's only because there is a lot of information about depression and social anxiety. As one of the most common mental health concerns, depression has very serious consequences for those who struggle with the disorder. Suicide is a grim consequence. Prolonged depression can also lead to medical-related illnesses and disease, such as diabetes and heart disease among others.

For the person who is challenged every day with depression, or the person who suffers severe anxiety when forced to interact with others, this book provides hope and encouragement in the knowledge that they are not alone. The information in this book illustrates that there are many ways to take control and manage their depression. It points out that there are options in therapy, in lifestyle choices, and in finding a way past the anxiety and emotional darkness.

For the family or friend of a person who is diagnosed with depression, this book offers insight and perspectives into these mental health diagnoses. With this knowledge comes the possibility that family and friends can provide the support and understanding to see their loved one through this tough struggle.

Lastly, if you enjoyed this book I ask that you please take the time to review it on Audible.com. Your honest feedback would be greatly appreciated.

Thank you

Now, I would like to share with you a free sneak peek to another one of my books that I think you will really enjoy. The book is called "Self Compassion: The Mindful Path to Understand your Emotions" by Kirstin Germer, Christopher Neff and it's A Practical Guide to Learn the Proven Power of Self-Acceptance, Self-Criticism, Self-Awareness and Mindfulness. You will also learn how to be Kind to Yourself and Move On.

Enjoy!

Introduction

Fostering a sense of self-compassion and self-acceptance can be challenging even for a healthy and well-rounded adult. Despite how important these two characteristics are, very few people are taught about how to utilize them in their personal lives. Instead, we are often taught to be hard on ourselves, push ourselves as far as we can, and demand the maximum results out of our efforts. While challenging yourself to achieve substantial growth is valuable, pushing yourself to the point where it becomes self-sabotaging is not a positive habit to support.

If you truly want to achieve all of the success that you desire in life, you need to have a clear understanding of your mental wellbeing and around how you can support it so that you can improve your chances of succeeding. Without a strong mindset to back them up, most people will fail to achieve their desired level of success because despite having the best of intentions, they will struggle to keep themselves focused and motivated. Through the emotional and mental self-sabotaging behaviors such as having an overly harsh inner critic or trying to push through challenging emotions without acknowledging their purpose or healing them, they will simply burn out and fail to thrive.

As you listen through this book, realize that you are going to be granted every single tool you need to begin developing the skills to become more self-compassionate and self-accepting. From identifying how to feel your emotions and develop a relationship to building a productive mindfulness and self-awareness practice, everything is devoted to helping you motivate yourself in a healthy way. The tools in this book will not encourage or motivate you to become complacent, lose focus, or stop aiming for your dreams with any less intensity than you already have been. Instead, they will support you in having a stronger focus on how you can achieve your goals without compromising your inner sense of wellbeing. As a result, all of the success that you earn in your life will feel far more meaningful and positive.

If self-compassion has been particularly challenging for you until now, or if the concept itself seems foreign, I encourage you to really set the intention to approach this book and the subjects within it with an open mind. You will get the most out of each chapter and all of the tools provided if you give yourself permission to see things from a new perspective at least for the duration of this book. Fully embrace the practice of not only learning about and understanding these concepts and tools but actually working towards putting them into practice in your life as well. As you begin to see just how powerful they are and how they support you in moving forward towards a more positive future, you will quickly begin to realize why they matter so much.

Lastly, there is one major concept that you need to realize before you begin listening this book. That is — self-compassion is an act of self-care, but it is also a tool that is learned through personal development practices. You are not going to be able to achieve self-compassion all in one attempt, nor will you truly be able to measure or grade yourself on the level of self-compassion that you currently have or that you develop. While there are ways for you to track your improvements and we will go into detail on those ways later, you need to understand that this practice is solely about helping yourself feel better and feel more positive in your approach to life. By allowing yourself to embody that balance, you will begin to feel far more peaceful overall.

Now, if you are ready to embark on the next chapter of your journey in self-development, it is time that you begin! Remember, self-compassion is a powerful tool for you to equip yourself with, so approach this book as open-mindedly as you possibly can. And of course, enjoy the process!

Chapter 1: Understanding the Self

Your Self or your identity is an important element of who you are. When you consider who you are, the illusion that you come up with is how you identify yourself. Although we tend to believe that our selves are an inherent part of who we are and that our personal beliefs over ourselves are finite and final, the reality is that who we are and who we think we are, typically reflect two entirely different people. Many people fail to realize that there is a difference and often find themselves genuinely believing that they are the person whom they envision in their minds and that there is no other alternative or option. As a result, they may end up developing a highly toxic, unrealistic, and self-sabotaging image or belief around who they are.

Realizing that who you truly are and who you think you are is two different people can come as a sense of relief to many. When you discover that there is a good chance that you do not actually align with the images or beliefs you have created, you realize that there is an opportunity for you to see yourself in a new light. You may even get the opportunity to start seeing yourself more clearly for who you really are, rather than for the illusion that you have been holding onto in your mind. In fact, by detaching from the strict identity you have held onto in your mind, you can give yourself the opportunity to begin experiencing far more compassion towards yourself in your life.

Identity is a rather complex topic that extends far beyond the image we carry of ourselves and the image that other's carry. In fact, there is an entire psychological study devoted to understanding identity and your sense of self and helping you discover exactly "who" you are. This field of study is known as social science and is comprised of psychologists and researchers who are actively seeking to understand identity to an even deeper level and get a clear sense of what makes a person's identity. Because there are so many different levels of identity, the study itself is quite expansive and continues to discover what one's true identity is versus the way they identify themselves and the way others identify them. In the following sections, you are going to get a deeper insight into what your sense of self truly is, how it is made up, and how your sense of self impacts the way you live your life.

Discovering the Multiple Selves

There are two ways that people have multiple sense of self. The first way that you can experience multiple senses of self comes from how you interact with the people around you and the identity you possess around these people. For example, the self you are around your friends is likely quite different from the self you are around your family or your co-workers. Your environment is a huge factor in which role you will play, depending on where you are and who you are actively surrounded by. The second way that you experience multiple social selves is determined between the way you perceive yourself and the way others perceive you. Since everyone has had their own unique interactions and experiences with you, it is not unreasonable to realize that everyone sees you slightly different from how others see you. For example, your best friend may see you completely different from how your other friends may see you, or your Grandma may carry a completely different belief of who you are compared to the rest of the world. The relationship that people share with you, the experiences that you share together, and their perception of you and of people in general will all impact how people identify you. As a result, you actually have multiple identities – and no, that does not mean that you are having an identity crisis or that you have something wrong with you. It is actually entirely normal to have many identities.

When it comes to identifying yourself, you must realize that on a psychological front, you are not identifying yourself as one person inhabiting one body. You are identifying yourself based on the actual identity that you carry or the characteristics and personality traits that you are perceived to have. Your "self" is the conscious aspect of you that interacts with the world around you, communicates with other people, and shares experiences with others. Although there is no scientific evidence that proves that there is an out-of-body "self," most psychologists believe that the self is not attached to or identified by a person's body. Instead, it is the dimension of you that exists in your mind or the aspects of you that make up "who" you are beyond your physical and biological self.

This part of yourself that is not defined by your body or biology is typically described in three related but separable domains when it comes to psychological understanding. This means that there are three elements that coincide to make up your "self" or your identity. The first domain is known as your experiential self which is also known as the 'theatre of consciousness.' This part of yourself is identified as your first-person sense of being or how you personally experience the world around you. This part of yourself remains consistent over periods of time which results in psychologists believing that it is very closely linked to your memory. The second part of your identity is what is known as your private self-consciousness. This is your inner narrator or the voice that verbally narrates what is happening in your life to you privately within your mind. When you are reading, learning, or interpreting the world around you, this voice is actively narrating how you are interpreting that information and what sense you are making of it. This is the part of you that carries your beliefs and values about how the world works. Neuroscientist Antonio Damasio calls your private self-consciousness your autobiographical self because it is regularly narrating your autobiography in your mind. The third and final dimension of your identity is your public self or your persona. This is the image that you attempt to project to others through your actions, attitudes, behaviors, and words. This is the part of your self that other people interact with and see which results in this being the part of yourself that people generate perceptions around. It is through your persona that people determine what your identity is according to them and their own understanding.

With all that being said, the multiple selves that you embody comes from the persona that you share with others. People will then generate perceptions around who you are, what your identity is, and how they feel about that. It is through this persona that people will decide if they can relate to you, if they like you, and anything else relating to how they feel about you. In realizing that people generate their perceptions of you based off of one single aspect of who you truly are, it helps you realize that their perspective is not accurate. In fact, neither is yours. No one, including yourself, *truly* knows who you actually are. Everything is just generated based on beliefs, values, perspectives, and understandings that have been accumulated through varying life experiences.

Relationship with Ourselves

The relationship that you share with yourself often develops somewhere between the first and second dimensions of your identity. The way you interpret and interact with the world around you, combined with your beliefs and values helps you generate a sort of self-awareness that allows you to begin determining what you believe your identity is. Again, just like with other people, your identity is largely based off of your perception and understanding of the world around you and how it works. Even if your own perception is rarely accurate when compared to who you actually are which is a unique blend of all three layers of your dimensional identity.

Because your relationship with yourself is largely defined by your beliefs and values and your ability to live in alignment with them or not, it is easy to realize that how you identify yourself can be easily shifted based on your perceptions. If you carry certain core beliefs about how people should live, for example, and you are not living in alignment with those beliefs, then you may generate a perception that identifies you as someone who is bad or unworthy. You might relate yourself to the identities you have mentally designed for other people in society who you believe to be bad too which can result in you seeing yourself in an extremely negative light. If you carry certain core beliefs about how people should live and you *are* living in alignment with them, you may praise yourself and see yourself as good and special. You might then find yourself relating more to people in society who you see as good and positive, thus allowing you to cast yourself in a positive light.

The reality is that none of us are truly inherently good or bad, we are all just perceiving, experiencing, and responding to the world around us. Generating internal images of what is positive and what is not only results in you setting standards for yourself on how you should behave. If these standards are beyond what you can reasonably achieve or do not align with what you genuinely want in life, then you may find yourself adhering to beliefs and values that are actually rather destructive. Instead of helping you live a life of contentment and satisfaction, you may find these beliefs leading to you constantly feeling incapable and under confident. As a result, your relationship with yourself may deteriorate because the way in which you view yourself is not reasonable or compassionate.

Everyone Has Their Own Filters and Explanatory Styles

To help you develop your understanding of how your perception of yourself varies from other's perception of you, let's discuss personal filters and explanatory styles. Understanding why everyone has such different views of the world allows you to have a stronger understanding as to why there are so many aspects of your identity based on your own personas and the way that people perceive them and you. The concept of personal filters and explanatory styles is simple. A personal filter is how you see the world and your explanatory style is how you explain it to yourself and to others.

Every single person has a unique filter and explanatory style that is based on their own unique experiences in life. All of the interactions they have had, the situations they have encountered, and things they have been told by the people around them shape the way that they view life itself. How each of these small yet impactful things come together will shape how each person perceives the world around them, others that cohabit the planet with them, and themselves. So, for example, if someone along the way has learned that not washing your dishes every day is a sign of laziness and ignorance, then that person is going to believe that anyone who leaves dishes in the sink overnight is somehow "bad," including themselves.

The foundation of a person's filters and explanatory styles are rooted in childhood when a child is not yet able to generate their own independent thoughts and beliefs. Until we are six years old, our ability to critically think about things and generate our own opinions independent of the opinions of others is virtually non-existent so we absorb everything we learn. This means that anything your parents said, people around you were saying, or you were shown through other's behaviors and actions were anchored into your mind as the foundation of your personal beliefs and values. Even though you gained the capacity to think critically and start generating your own opinions around six years old, you were still actively internalizing what everyone told you because, in most cases, no one ever taught you otherwise. As a result, you likely have many different beliefs and values that stemmed in your childhood which have gone on to impact you for years to come. In fact, these very beliefs and values are believed to make up a lot of what your autobiographical-self narrates to yourself on a daily basis, thus shaping the way you see yourself. See, who you think you are may not even be an accurate reflection of how *you* think, it may actually be an internalization based on the beliefs and values you were taught by people as you were growing up.

Since every single person will hear different things throughout their lives even if they are raised in similar environments, the way that every person views and interprets the world around them varies. Even siblings will grow up to have different perceptions and beliefs based on the way that they have internalized the beliefs they heard and were shown throughout their lifetimes. It is through this process that each person develops their own personal filters and explanatory styles for how they interpret and explain the world around them. Because of this, we can conclude that any beliefs that you have around who you are and any beliefs that others have around who you are do not actually define who you truly are. Instead, they define the belief systems that you have established throughout your life until this point.

When you realize that your beliefs are what shape your *perception* of your identity and not your identity itself, it becomes a lot easier for you to have compassion for yourself. You begin to realize that how you see yourself is not necessarily a true reflection of who you are, but instead a way that you have been lead to view yourself. This view was designed to support you in feeling connected to your 'tribe' or family and community, but in some cases, it can become destructive and result in you feeling deeply disconnected from yourself. When that happens, realizing that you are not inherently 'bad' or 'wrong' because you do not feel like you fit in makes it a lot easier for you to have compassion for your feelings and for the experiences you are going through. As a result, healing from these painful emotions and moving forward into a more self-compassionate and self-loving future becomes a lot easier for you.

Thank you, this preview in now finished.

If you enjoyed this preview of my book "The Mindful Path to Self-Compassion" by Frank Steven, be sure to check out the full book on Amazon.com

Thank you.

The Adult ADHD & ADD Solution

Discover How to Restore Attention and Reduce Hyperactivity in Just 14 Days. The Complete Guide for Diagnosed Children and Parents

By Julia Kruger

© Copyright 2018 - All rights reserved.

The content contained within this book may not be reproduced, duplicated or transmitted without direct written permission from the author or the publisher.

Under no circumstances will any blame or legal responsibility be held against the publisher, or author, for any damages, reparation, or monetary loss due to the information contained within this book. Either directly or indirectly.

Legal Notice:

This book is copyright protected. This book is only for personal use. You cannot amend, distribute, sell, use, quote or paraphrase any part, or the content within this book, without the consent of the author or publisher.

Disclaimer Notice:

Please note the information contained within this document is for educational and entertainment purposes only. All effort has been executed to present accurate, up to date, and reliable, complete information. No warranties of any kind are declared or implied. Readers acknowledge that the author is not engaging in the rendering of legal, financial, medical or professional advice. The content within this book has been derived from various sources. Please consult a licensed professional before attempting any techniques outlined in this book.

By reading this document, the reader agrees that under no circumstances is the author responsible for any losses, direct or indirect, which are incurred as a result of the use of information contained within this document, including, but not limited to, — errors, omissions, or inaccuracies.

Table of Contents

Chapter 1: What is ADD & ADHD?..125
   Introduction to ADD & ADHD..125
   What Causes ADHD? 125
   Which Groups Are At Risk? 126
      Types of ADHD...127
      Hyperactivity-Impulsivity ADHD Type 128
      Managing Hyperactivity-Impulsivity ADHD 128
      Inattentive ADHD..129
      Dealing with Inattentive ADHD 131
      Combination ADHD 132
      Test Your Type of ADHD 134
   Common Misconceptions about ADHD 134
      Only Kids can have ADHD 135
      ADHD Only Exists in Your Head 135
      ADHD Signifies Laziness and Lack of Motivation 136
      ADHD is Over-Diagnosed.......................................136
      You Must be Hyperactive to Have ADHD 136
      If You Can Concentrate on Some Tasks, You Do Not Have ADHD 137
      Medicine Can Treat ADHD.......................................137
      ADHD Is not a Real Medical Condition 138
      ADHD Results from Bad Parenting............................. 138
      ADHD Kids Can Concentrate if they Try Harder to Pay Attention 138
      ADHD Individuals Cannot Focus 139
      Everyone who has ADHD is Hyperactive....................139
      ADHD Only Affects Males 139
      ADHD is a Learning Disability 140
      Kids With ADHD Will Eventually Outgrow It 141

Chapter 2: Child with ADHD 142
   What Causes ADHD among Kids? 144
      Environmental Factors 144
      Brain Injury...145
      Sugar and Food Additives.......................................145
      Genetic Causes 145

Symptoms of a Child With ADHD.. 146
Criteria for Diagnosing ADHD in Kids................................147
Diagnosing ADHD in Kids.. 148
    Who Should Diagnose ADHD in Kids? 149
Which Other Disorders Accompany ADHD Among Kids? 152
    Learning Disabilities..152
    Tourette Syndrome 152
    Oppositional Defiant Disorder 153
    Conduct Disorder...153
    Anxiety and Depression...153
    Bipolar Disorder 154

Chapter 3: Attention Deficit Hyperactivity Disorder in Adults 155
    Symptoms of Adult ADHD 156
        Hyperactivity-Impulsivity Symptoms in Adults 156
        Inattentive ADHD Symptoms in Adults........................157
    The Appearance of ADHD Symptoms Amongst Adults ... 157
    Diagnosing ADHD in Adults 158
    Couples with ADHD 159
        Couples' Expectation Guide on ADHD Marriage.......... 160
        ADHD at the Workplace 166

Chapter 4: Medical and Treatment Guidance for ADHD..... 171
    Medication for ADHD Types.. 171
        Medication for Hypersensitive-Impulsive ADHD Type 171
        Medication for Inattentive ADHD...................................172
        Non-Stimulant Medication for ADHD 173
    Treatment in Kids..174
        Medical Interventions for ADHD Kids..........................174
    Treatment of ADHD in Adults 184
        Therapy 184
        Risks of Untreated Adult ADHD 186
How Long Should ADHD Medication be Administered? .187
Should Patients Consider Psychotherapy? 188
ADHD Coaching 188
Can ADHD Be Treated Without Drugs? 189
Alternative Interventions to Medicines and Therapy...... 190

    Sleep 190
    Exercise 190
    Meditation and Mindfulness 191
  Recommended Food & Supplements to help with ADHD 193
    Supplements Used to Manage ADHD Symptoms 193
    Herbs for ADHD 195
    ADHD Diets 195
Chapter 5: ADHD and Other Mental Disorders 197
  ADHD With Learning Disabilities in a Child 197
    What Are Some of the Most Common Learning
    Disabilities? 198
    What is the Connection Between Learning Difficulties
    and ADHD? 199
    Tips to Overcome Learning Difficulties and ADHD 199
  ADHD with Autism Spectrum Disorder in a Child and
  an Adult 200
    What is the Difference Between ADHD and Autism? .. 201
    Diagnosing ASD and ADHD 202
    Tips to Overcome ASD and ADHD Comorbidity 202
  ADHD With Anxiety 203
    Differentiating Between Anxiety and ADHD 204
    What is the Connection Between Anxiety and ADHD? 205
    Tips to Overcome ADHD and Anxiety Disorder
    Comorbidity 206
  ADHD With Depression 209
    What is the Link Between ADHD and Depression? 210
    What Are the Distinguishing Symptoms Between
    ADHD and Depression? 211
  Tips to Overcome Depression With ADHD 212
  ADHD With Bipolar Disorder 214
    Managing ADHD With Bipolar Disorder 215
Conclusion 217
The Mind with Cognitive Behavioral Therapy 218

Congratulations on purchasing The Adult ADHD & ADD Solution, and thank you for doing so!

The following chapters will discuss how to Overcome ADHD as a Parent. The Effects on Marriage and Relationships. Best ways to Parenting kids and teenagers with ADHD. The information found in this book will best explore the diets and treatments in order to Restore Focus and attention.

Thanks again for choosing this book! Every effort was made to ensure it is full of as much useful information as possible.

Please enjoy!

Chapter 1: What is ADD & ADHD?

Introduction to ADD & ADHD

ADHD (attention deficit hyperactivity disorder) is among the most prevalent childhood disorders. This learning disorder was formerly known as ADD (attention deficit disorder) and according to the Center for Disease Control and Prevention, more than 6.4 million children have been diagnosed with it. The disorder has an effect on the behavior, learning ability, and emotions of those who are affected. In as much as ADHD is most prevalent among children, it is also common in adults. Those who are affected by this condition in adulthood always start experiencing its symptoms in childhood.

The rate of ADHD prevalence amongst school-going children is estimated to be 11%. Most cases end up being diagnosed because ADHD typically overlaps other behavioral disorders that weaken individuals' cognitive skills, thus making it difficult for clinicians to categorize whatever they see. It has largely been claimed that ADHD is a modern disorder owing to the fact that it has only been on the rise in recent years.

Pinpointing the rate of ADHD prevalence in all demographics of the population remains a grey area because there are glaring discrepancies among people who are diagnosed with it. The situation is compounded further by the fact that mental health specialists use varying criteria to diagnose the disorder. Besides this, cultural factors pertaining to what should be considered normal behavior varies from one place to another. Behaviors that point towards the positive diagnosis of ADHD in some places could be considered normal in other regions.

What Causes ADHD?

Even though no one can explicitly point out the exact cause of ADHD, it has been proven that various factors play a contributory role. Since ADHD symptoms- inattention, hyperactivity and/or impulsivity affect a child's or adult's ability to get along with others, many people assume that the behavior exhibited by such individuals is as a result of poor discipline, a chaotic upbringing, or even too much TV watching. This is skewed thinking since ADHD traits run in families. Up to half of adults who have ADHD will end up having kids with the disorder. Generally, there are generic traits which get passed down from an ADHD adult to his/her kids. If an adult has ADHD, there's a 50% chance that his/her kids will have it. Likewise, there's a 30% chance of ADHD being present in a younger sibling if an older sibling has it. Nevertheless, the manner in which ADHD is inherited is complex since it cannot be linked to one genetic fault.

Research also indicates that ADHD can be caused by an individual's brain structure and function. There are various possible differences in the brain of individuals who have ADHD and those that do not have the condition. Even so, the exact difference isn't clear. For instance, studies on brain scans have revealed that certain parts of the human brain may be smaller in individuals who have ADHD compared to those who don't have the condition. Likewise, other parts may be abnormally larger. Other studies have also suggested that individuals who have ADHD tend to have an imbalance as far as the level of neurotransmitters in their brain is concerned. In other cases, these neurotransmitters do not function properly. Pregnancy problems are also likely to lead to ADHD. Children who have low birth weight and those who are born prematurely are likely to have ADHD.

Which Groups Are At Risk?

Researchers believe that certain groups are at more risk of having ADHD. This includes babies who are born prematurely before the 37th week of pregnancy, and those who have a low birth weight. Similarly individuals who have epilepsy are at high risk of also having ADHD. Those who have brain injury that occurred either in the womb during pregnancy or after a severe impact on the head later in life are also at a high risk of suffering from ADHD.

Mothers who endure difficult pregnancies are also likely to give birth to kids who are at a high risk of having the disorder. Likewise, kids who have head injuries at the brain's frontal lobe are also at a high risk of being diagnosed with ADHD. Toxins also raise the chances of having ADHD with studies indicating that pregnant mothers who drink alcohol or smoke are at a high risk of giving birth to children with ADHD. Likewise, exposure to PCBs, pesticides, and lead during pregnancy also increases the chances of having ADHD. Such toxins typically interfere with kids' brain development.

Types of ADHD

The Diagnostic and Statistical Manual of Mental Disorders indicates that there are three main types of ADHD. These are:

- Inattentive ADHD
- Hyperactive-Impulsive ADHD
- Combination Type ADHD

People who have ADHD may show signs and symptoms of being consistently inattentive just the same way that they are likely to be more impulsive and hyperactive than their peers of the same age. Some have a combination of inattentive and impulsive behaviors.

The predominantly hyperactive-impulsive ADHD patients do not portray significant inattention. On the other hand, predominantly inattentive ADHD patients do not exhibit notable hyperactive or impulsive behavior. The combination type displays behaviors that relate to both inattentiveness and hyperactivity.

Hyperactivity-Impulsivity ADHD Type

Individuals who have this type of ADHD often experience immense hyperactivity, which makes them want to be always "on the go." You will see a kid dashing around, talking incessantly, or even playing with whatever they come across. Staying still to concentrate on simple tasks is difficult for such individuals since their mind is always wandering. You will see them squirming in their seats or fidgeting with objects within their reach, or just roaming around the room. Hyperactive adults tend to feel internally restless, something that leads them to undertake several tasks at once. If not well managed, they end up failing in all these tasks because none of them tends to be given the attention that it deserves. Other signs of hyperactivity-impulsivity in kids include blurting out answers even before they hear the whole question, and having difficulty taking turns or waiting in line. Children who have the hyperactive-impulsive ADHD type tend to be disruptive to the extent that they make learning difficult, not only for themselves but also for others.

Managing Hyperactivity-Impulsivity ADHD

Handling someone who has hyperactivity-impulsivity ADHD can be difficult because such individuals always seem to have boundless energy. More often than less, those who have this type of ADHD are seen to be overly aggressive and unruly due to the impulsive nature of their actions and social interactions. Even though these individuals can be sensitive to other people's feelings, their good qualities tend to be eclipsed by their relatively poor impulse control and ability to self-regulate.

To manage hyperactivity-impulsivity ADHD among kids, you should put in place impulse control measures. This may include posting classroom routines and rules to let them know what is expected of them. These rules also act as a constant visual reminder of what they should do at all times. Hyperactivity-impulsivity ADHD can also be managed by preparing kids for any transitions. In most cases, kids suffering from this type of ADHD have meltdowns when exposed to transitions in between activities. Warning them prior to making changes to their schedules gives them time to end one activity and embark on the next one.

When handling kids who have hyperactivity-impulsivity ADHD, you should always be prepared for hyperactive behavior and impulsive reactions. Once you know that a situation can set off impulsive reactions, always have a plan to keep the impulses in check. For instance, assigning coaches to kids suffering from this type of ADHD will help them maintain their self-control and stay focused.

Inattentive ADHD

Those who suffer from this type of ADHD typically have a hard time when it comes to keeping their mind focused on one activity. They tend to get bored easily and switch off their minds from whatever is happening around them. When engaging in activities that they enjoy, such kids won't have any trouble paying attention. Nonetheless, focusing on their attention on deliberate action is difficult. It even gets harder for them to complete tasks or learn something new due to lapses in concentration. Needless to say, kids are natural dreamers. It isn't unusual to find a kid staring into space or lost in thought. Failure to complete tasks assigned to them may ultimately lead to frustration for both child and parent. Your kid could be having inattentive ADHD if he/she constantly finds it difficult to focus.

Inattentive ADHD is sometimes referred to as Attentive Deficit Disorder (ADD). Sometimes, this type of ADHD is mistaken for mood or anxiety disorder, especially among adults. In children, it typically gets mistaken for a learning disorder. It is easy to ignore this behavioral disorder and, consequently, kids who are affected seldom get the treatment that they require. In the long run, this may lead to undue shame and apathy, which can last throughout an individual's life.

Children who have the inattention type of ADHD are rarely hyperactive or impulsive. Nonetheless, they have difficulties when it comes to paying attention. In most cases, they will appear confused, "spacey," slow, or lethargic. They also tend to experience difficulties in processing information as accurately and quickly as other kids. When given oral instructions, they find it hard to process what is required of them. As a result, they end up making frequent mistakes.

The American Psychiatric Association has a diagnostic manual, which lists 9 common symptoms of inattentive ADHD. When diagnosing inattentive ADHD, at least 6 of these symptoms ought to be present, and should also be significantly disruptive. This will merit the diagnosis of inattentive ADHD. Kids are deemed to have inattentive ADHD if they:

- often fail to pay close attention to detail, and consequently end up making careless mistakes in their schoolwork and other activities they engage in.
- often get distracted and are thus unable to concentrate on tasks or activities.
- often have trouble when it comes to following instructions. This makes it difficult for them to complete

their chores and any other duties that may be allocated to them.

- often find it difficult to organize tasks and activities.
- often avoid undertaking tasks, or are reluctant to partake in tasks that require sustained mental effort.
- tend to lose items such as notebooks, which are needed to complete tasks assigned to them.
- are forgetful when it comes to their schedules.

Dealing with Inattentive ADHD

In the event that your child is diagnosed with inattentive ADHD, all is not lost, since you can still improve his/her ability to concentrate on tasks and activities. Generally, a combination of therapy and medication works best. You can undertake behavioral therapy yourself to mitigate inattentive ADHD. Parenting tactics that can be incorporated when offering behavioral therapy to kids with inattentive ADHD may include setting up a reward system for good behavior, and withholding privileges or taking away rewards in an effort to deal with undesirable behavior. Such methods can be used by teachers, parents, and counselors, to help kids who have inattentive ADHD stay on track.

Since children who suffer from inattentive ADHD are forgetful, you can keep them up to speed with tasks that they are supposed to do by creating to-do lists. These lists could contain household and school chores as examples. Posting the lists in places where the kids can easily see them, will keep them apprised with whatever they are supposed to do. It is also advisable that you break down projects into small tasks. Bite-sizing projects will go a long way in preventing kids from getting bored. Rather than telling them to do their homework, for instance, you can request them to read one chapter of their language book. This makes the task at hand appear less mentally strenuous and will give them the impetus to undertake them.

To enhance the concentration span of kids with inattentive ADHD, you should always give them clear instructions. Whatever instructions that you give to them ought to be simple and easy to decipher. Any complexities are likely to cause such kids to switch off their brains, even before they undertake the task at hand. In addition, you should get them into a routine, since a sense of order goes a long way in helping inattentive ADHD kids stay focused. Following a known routine on a daily basis will let them know what is expected of them. You should similarly endeavor to minimize distractions around inattentive ADHD kids since they tend to snap out of concentration even with the slightest disruption. At home, turn off the TV, computers, and video games when the kids are undertaking a task. Likewise, ask their teachers to move them away from doors or windows at school so that they do not get distracted by activities happening outside the classroom. You should also offer rewards whenever inattentive ADHD kids finish tasks on time. Making them feel appreciated will spur them to be more attentive when undertaking future tasks.

Combination ADHD

Combination type ADHD manifests itself when both hyperactivity-impulsivity and inattention are present. In this case, those affected will have the inability to focus at some point and likewise; they will also be unable to stay still at another point. Most kids experience the combination type of ADHD and this is perhaps why the behavioral disorder is rarely diagnosed and treated during childhood. Most of us think that it is normal for kids to experience bouts of hyperactivity and impulsivity followed by inattention.

When someone exhibits 6 or more symptoms of either inattentive or hyperactivity-impulsivity ADHD, chances are high that he/she could be suffering from combination type ADHD. Therefore, a doctor will look out for symptoms of both inattentiveness and hyperactivity when diagnosing combination type ADHD. The diagnosis of this disorder typically involves undertaking a medical examination to rule out other behavioral disorders, such as anxiety. A medical examination may also involve surveys to establish your child's behavior and interaction with others.

Combination type ADHD treatments involve both medication and therapy to improve the child's attention, besides lowering his/her hyperactivity or impulsivity. Psycho-stimulants may be used to ease common behavioral symptoms of combined ADHD, thus making it easier for kids to focus on their everyday tasks.

The symptoms that kids exude are what help determine the type of ADHD that they are suffering from. Since symptoms exhibited by patients may be caused by a different behavioral disorder, it is advisable that patients undergo a thorough diagnosis to determine the type of ADHD that they are suffering from. ADHD symptoms tend to appear over a long period. More often than less, symptoms of hyperactivity and impulsiveness precede those that characterize inattentive ADHD. Besides this, different ADHD symptoms emerge in different settings. For instance, a kid who cannot sit still or portrays disruptive behavior in school is more likely to be noticed than an inattentive daydreamer within the same setting. Likewise, impulsive kids who typically act before thinking are said to have discipline issues while those who exhibit passive behavior are likely to be seen as being merely unmotivated or lazy.

Such prognosis is wrong, considering the fact that both sets of kids show behaviors that point towards different types of ADHD. Generally, all kids sometimes get restless, just the same way that they act without thinking at times. Likewise, kids sometimes daydream their time away. Exhibiting any of these signs alone doesn't show that a kid has ADHD. That can only be the case if a child's distractibility, poor concentration, hyperactivity, or impulsivity, begins to affect their school performance, social relationships, and overall behavior. When this happens, ADHD may be suspected. Since ADHD symptoms vary from one setting to another, diagnosing the condition, therefore, isn't easy.

Test Your Type of ADHD

Just like it is the case with most behavioral disorders, there is no single test that can be exclusively used to diagnose ADHD in both kids and adults. A combination of psychological tests and rating scales to determine the symptoms of ADHD will help you determine whether or not you are affected by the condition. When testing for your type of ADHD, you should first know the symptoms of each. If you exhibit at least six symptoms of hyperactivity-impulsivity, you could have this type of ADHD. Likewise, you could have the inattentive type of ADHD if you have at least six symptoms that characterize the disorder. If you have combination type ADHD, you will certainly exhibit symptoms of both hyperactivity-impulsivity and inattentiveness.

Common Misconceptions about ADHD

A lot of myths and misconceptions about ADHD exist in the public domain. Much of the misinformation about ADHD pertains to its causes, diagnosis, and treatment. The following are some of these common myths.

Only Kids can have ADHD

This is perhaps the most peddled misconception as far as ADHD is concerned. Contrary to what many people think, ADHD affects both children and adults. The misconception that only kids can be affected by this behavioral disorder, is attributed to the fact that its symptoms ought to be exhibited by the age of 7 years so that the criteria for diagnosis is met. A large number of those who are affected remain undiagnosed until they reach adulthood. In some cases, ADHD is diagnosed in adults only after diagnosis has been made on their own kids.

A number of adults only recognize that they have ADHD traits after learning more about it. Such a realization may lead you to reflect on your own childhood and recall whatever struggles you had in school and problems with inattention, that weren't ever treated. You should keep in mind that up to 70% of kids who have ADHD will continue exhibiting symptoms of the conditions up to the time they reach adulthood.

Hyperactive behaviors that are common in children who have ADHD may decrease as they age, but nonetheless, ADHD symptoms, such as inattention, restlessness, and distractibility, may persist into adulthood. If left untreated, adult ADHD often leads to chronic problems at work and in social relationships. It can lead to more serious issues such as depression, anxiety, and substance abuse.

ADHD Only Exists in Your Head

Hypothetically, ADHD is a mental issue, because certain brain regions of patients who have the disorder fail to synchronize properly. This has led many to believe that people only use ADHD as a justification for not focusing on completing their tasks. Nonetheless, this isn't the case. It goes without saying that the brains of individuals with ADHD work differently from those of people who do not have the condition. In the former, the medial prefrontal cortex and the posterior cingulate cortex don't match up, thus leading to concentration issues. This alone proves that ADHD isn't just a typical mental issue used as an excuse for lack of focus when undertaking tasks.

ADHD Signifies Laziness and Lack of Motivation

This misconception is a typical response to behaviors exhibited by kids struggling with inattentive ADHD. In most cases, such kids are seen to be lazy and unmotivated because we fail to look at the underlying cause of their lethargic behavior. Your kid could be finding it difficult to undertake tasks that require continued mental exertion, not because he/she is lazy, but due to ADHD. Therefore, this disorder should not be used as an excuse to label someone as lazy or unmotivated. Besides this, ADHD has nothing to do with an individual's intellectual ability. Plenty of individuals who struggle with the condition are extremely creative and sharp; they only work in a manner that is different from others.

ADHD is Over-Diagnosed

This misconception is informed by the fact that the number of diagnosed ADHD cases has been on the rise in the recent past. Although the number of reported ADHD diagnoses has increased significantly, it shouldn't be misconstrued to mean that the condition is over-diagnosed. It simply means that many people are waking up to the realization that ADHD is real. Consequently, more people are seeking diagnosis and treatment thus the increase in reported cases.

You Must be Hyperactive to Have ADHD

This misconception perhaps stems from the "hyperactive" part of the disorder's title Many people think that you only need to be hyperactive for you to have ADHD. Such individuals tend to forget that predominant inattentiveness and a combination of inattentiveness and hyperactivity also signify someone as having ADHD. Since the inattentive type of ADHD is less disruptive, you may think that those affected do not suffer from ADHD. Likewise, having trouble focusing on tasks doesn't automatically mean that you have ADHD.

If You Can Concentrate on Some Tasks, You Do Not Have ADHD

The fact that ADHD is largely an "attention deficit" disorder makes it quite confusing when you see someone with it concentrating intently on a task. It seems even more fitting to describe the disorder as a condition that forces individuals to have trouble regulating their attention. In as much as those who are affected by ADHD have significant problems focusing their attention on completing tasks, they still maintain the ability to focus on activities that are stimulating. This is known as hyperfocus.

Medicine Can Treat ADHD

Medications, including stimulants and non-stimulants, play an important role in curbing common ADHD symptoms. A combination of treatment goes a long way in manage ADHD. Nonetheless, medicines shouldn't be used in isolation, since behavioral therapy and DIY strategies, such as leaving reminders and notes around the house to keep you up to speed with tasks that you are supposed to undertake, play an important part in minimizing the effects of ADHD.

In as much as medication is the most effective intervention against ADHD, it isn't the only intervention that works. Combining medication with cognitive and behavioral therapy will help quell the symptoms of ADHD. It is important for parents whose kids have ADHD to seek other alternatives which can help manage symptoms of the conditions.

Contrary to public perception, medications used in ADHD management do not cure the condition. Their purpose is to help control common ADHD symptoms. ADHD is a chronic behavioral disorder that doesn't go away it is only the symptoms that may lessen or change over time. Developing organizing and coping strategies will help manage and control the symptoms of ADHD.

ADHD Is not a Real Medical Condition

This is one of the most common ADHD myths that you will find out there. Many argue that ADHD is just a behavioral condition and not a medical condition. According to the <u>National Center for Disease Control</u> and the <u>American Psychiatric Association</u>, ADHD is a medical condition. It is hereditary in nature since one out of every four people who have ADHD has a parent who also has the condition. Similarly, imaging studies have shown that there is a difference in the brain development of kids who have ADHD and kids who do not have the condition.

ADHD Results from Bad Parenting

This is another common ADHD myth in the public domain. Generally, individuals who have ADHD tend to exhibit antisocial behavior. Many people end up believing that the cause of this behavior is bad parenting. It common for people to attribute inappropriate comments or constant fidgeting among individuals with ADHD, to poor parenting. Unbeknown to them, these are some of the standouts signs of ADHD and have nothing to do with parenting.

ADHD Kids Can Concentrate if they Try Harder to Pay Attention

Kids and adults who have ADHD often struggle to pay attention. Many people believe that the lack of attention is deliberate and that those with ADHD can concentrate if only they try or learn to pay attention. What many people don't know is the fact that ADHD patients often try as hard as "normal people" to pay attention. Telling individuals who have ADHD to focus is akin to asking a short-sighted person to look farther without wearing glasses.

Research indicates that there is a difference in the pathways of the brains kids and adults with ADHD. Generally, these pathways take longer to develop or may function less efficiently and therefore, such individuals end up experiencing concentration lapses.

ADHD Individuals Cannot Focus

Some people who tend to get easily distracted often have trouble shifting their attention from tasks that they enjoy the most. For instance, a child who is watching cartoons or playing with toys can be hyper-focused on that activity. This doesn't necessarily mean that such a child can pay better attention to tasks than kids who have ADHD. It's only a matter of interest in whatever activity that they are engaged in rather than an issue of hyperfocus or lack of focus.

Everyone who has ADHD is Hyperactive

It has long been believed that hyperactivity is the only symptom of ADHD. This is a flawed line of thought since not everyone who is hyperactive has ADHD. Likewise, not everyone who has ADHD is hyperactive. This highlights the importance of understanding the different ADHD types before making an assessment of an individual's behavior.

ADHD Only Affects Males

Needless to say, boys are at a higher risk of having ADHD compared to girls. However, this has been construed to mean that ADHD only affects males. Generally, girls can also have

ADHD only that it tends to be overlooked and thus remains undiagnosed. From a young age, society thinks it's normal for boys to be hyperactive, and girls to be less active. This could perhaps explain why many people have been led to believe that ADHD is a male affair. Attention issues tend to be different in boys than girls. Often, girls who have ADHD tend to have less difficulty when it comes to impulse and hyperactivity control. They are likely to seem more "day-dreamy" and out of touch with things happening around them.

As far as ADHD is concerned, girls generally tend to have less trouble than boys especially with hyperactivity. Nonetheless, this doesn't mean that they never experience hyperactivity. Instead, it will look different in them compared to boys. Girls often come across as being overly emotional or hypersensitive. Parents and teachers may notice them barging into conversations or even being a little more chatty than normal girls. For this reason, girls with ADHD are likely to fly under the radar.

ADHD is a Learning Disability

In as much as ADHD hinders the ability to pay attention and learn, it is a behavioral disorder and not a learning disability. It is only the main symptoms of ADHD that impact individuals' overall ability and capacity to learn. It goes without saying that kids can't do well in school or in their social interactions if they lack the ability to focus.

While ADHD only affects focus, learning disabilities tend to affect specific skills such as solving mathematical quizzes. The popularity of the myth that ADHD is a learning disability is attributed to the fact that most learning disabilities occur in comorbidity with ADHD. Similarly, the fact that ADHD is not a learning disability shouldn't mean that kids can't receive help. Devising an Individualized Educational Program can go a long way in helping ADHD kids learn just like other kids.

Kids With ADHD Will Eventually Outgrow It

ADHD is a lifelong disease, which nobody can outgrow. Many people tend to believe that they can overcome the condition as they grow older. Even though some of the symptoms of ADHD tend to change or disappear altogether as one grows older, it doesn't mean that the condition has disappeared.

As one grows older, he/she is likely to learn ways of managing ADHD symptoms. Many people look at this and conclude that the condition has been overcome. Those who have ADHD during childhood will continue having symptoms throughout their adolescence and adulthood. It is only that some of the symptoms may be subdued.

Chapter 2: Child with ADHD

This behavioral disorder is more common in kids than adults, thus making it necessary for parents to recognize the symptoms of ADHD. This will go a long way in helping them manage the condition in case their kids are affected. It is totally normal for kids to occasionally daydream in class, act impulsively, fidget at the dinner table, or even forget about their homework. What many parents do not understand is that the underlying cause of such behavior could be much deeper than what meets the eye. Impulsivity, hyperactivity, and inattention are some of the most notable signs of ADHD.

We have all encountered kids who cannot stay still, those who don't follow instructions, and those who always seem to be daydreaming. More often than less, such kids are deemed to be troublemakers, lazy, or undisciplined. The behaviors that such kids have are a pointer that they could be suffering from ADHD. Typically, ADHD symptoms in kids appear before they reach seven years. Nonetheless, the unpredictable nature of kids often makes it difficult to distinguish between those who are "normal" from those who are affected by attention deficit hyperactivity disorder.

It is generally advisable that you take a close look at your kid if he/she starts exhibiting a number of ADHD symptoms across different situations when playing, at home, and in school. It is only after you have understood the exact ADHD issue that your kid is struggling with, that you can work out a creative solution for remedying the disorder.

The stereotypical ADHD patients is an 8-year old kid who has the tendency to jump off from high points dangerously, or never even remembers to raise his/her hand while in class. In reality, only a few people who have ADHD fit this description.

Generally, kids who have the tendency to bounce off chairs or prank their playmates are usually the first ones to be evaluated for ADHD and to be diagnosed. On the other hand, those that have the tendency to have the tendency to wander off while in class often fly off the radar.

The National Institute of Mental Health points out that most inattention symptoms are less likely to be pinpointed by parents, medical professionals, and teachers. As a result, those who suffer from inattention ADHD rarely receive the treatment that they need. These kids often exhibit symptoms of academic frustration, undue shame due to poor academic and social performance, and apathy. These may last throughout their lifetime.

Often, inattention ADHD is regarded as spacey and apathetic behavior among kids, and mood disorders among adults. Individuals who suffer from inattention ADHD tend to lose focus when engaging in mentally exerting tasks. They are also forgetful, and have trouble listening. Kids who have inattention ADHD may rush through quizzes while missing questions whose answers they know, or they may even skip whole sections in their haste. This habit may persist until adulthood whereby adults who have ADHD often fail to proofread documents carefully at work. This way, they end up attracting unwanted embarrassment and attention.

Kids who have inattention ADHD similarly have a shorter attention span compared to other kids. They will submit unfinished classwork, incomplete reading assignments, or do house chores halfway. As they grow older and transition into adulthood, they will despise long work meetings more than their "normal" colleagues do. To sustain their attention during meetings, you will find them sipping coffee, chewing gum or standing up during meetings. In addition, they have poor listening skills besides lacking the ability to follow up on tasks.

What Causes ADHD among Kids?

Needless to say, one of the first questions that you will ask yourself when one of your kids has been diagnosed with ADHD is, "what went wrong?" In as much as we cannot explicitly pinpoint one factor that leads to ADHD, research indicates that the disorder is caused by a myriad of factors. There is little evidence to suggest that ADHD arises purely from either child-rearing methods or social factors. Most of the substantiated causes tend to fall within the realm of genetics and neurobiology. Nonetheless, this shouldn't mean that environmental factors cannot influence the severity of ADHD.

Parents need to focus on finding the best ways of helping their kids cope with ADHD, rather than trying to establish what caused the disorder in the first place. Scientists are still attempting to establish what really causes ADHD in an effort to find better ways of treating and even preventing the condition. They are similarly seeking to prove that ADHD doesn't result from the home environment but rather from biological factors. Such knowledge will relieve parents of the guilt that typically sets in once kids are diagnosed with ADHD.

Here are some of the causes of ADHD.

Environmental Factors

Research indicates that there's a link between cigarette smoking and alcohol consumption during pregnancy, and the occurrence of ADHD in the offspring. As a precaution, pregnant mothers are advised to refrain from cigarettes and alcohol use. A high lead level is another environmental factor that increases the risk of ADHD among kids. Despite the fact that lead isn't allowed in paint, it is still present in older buildings. When pre-school kids are exposed to chemical agents like lead, the risk of ADHD increases.

Brain Injury

One of the earliest theories that were advanced by scientists is that, just like other attention disorders; brain injury greatly contributes to ADHD. Notably, children who have been involved in accidents that eventually led to brain injury tend to have ADHD-like behaviors, including inattention. Nevertheless, it has been established that only an insignificant percentage of kids who have ADHD have suffered traumatic brain injuries in their lives.

Sugar and Food Additives

It has long been suggested that most attention disorders, including ADHD, are caused by the consumption of food additives and refined sugars. Other researchers claim that most ADHD symptoms are exacerbated by food additives and sugar. The National Institutes of Health even held a scientific conference to find consensus on this issue. Ultimately, it was established that diet restrictions only helped a paltry 5% of kids who have ADHD; most of them being young, pre-school children with food allergies.

Genetic Causes

Generally, most attention disorders run in families. Therefore, there is a possibility that ADHD is genetically-transmitted. Research indicates that up to 25% of close family members of kids who have ADHD also have the condition. On the flipside, the rate is only 5% in the general population. Studies among twins also show that there is a notable genetic influence in ADHD. There are ongoing studies that aim to pinpoint the exact genes that cause kids to be vulnerable to ADHD. In line with this, the Attention Deficit Hyperactivity Disorder Molecular Genetics Network was established to act as a platform for researchers to share findings pertaining to possible genetic influences as far as this behavioral disorder is concerned.

Symptoms of a Child With ADHD

When you think of ADHD in kids, what probably comes to mind is a picture of a beyond-control kid who is impulsive and disruptive to everything around them. Nevertheless, this isn't the only behavior that ADHD kids portray. Likewise, kids who always seem docile and uninterested in whatever is happening around them are not lazy or stupid.

ADHD is in kids is akin to a three-lane highway. Some kids who have the disorder will be hyperactive and impulsive at all times. You will see them bouncing off walls, fidgeting with things around them, and generally wanting to engage their seemingly endless energy in physical activities. Such kids similarly react to situations impulsively and will blurt out responses without taking a moment to think. Most times, these kids are seen to be rash, ill-disciplined, and generally unmanaged.

On the other hand, some kids who have ADHD will always seem to be inattentive and detached from events around them. You will find such kids staring blankly into space while in class, with their attention miles away. They hardly engage in social activities and they also find it difficult to complete tasks that are mentally draining. They also find it difficult to shift their attention from one activity to the next.

Inattentive ADHD kids are typically regarded to be lazy and uninterested. Other kids have a unique character that combines hyperactivity and impulsivity with inattentiveness. Kids that show these signs will be hyperactive and impulsive at one point and reclusive at some other point. When interacting with such kids, most of us may end up thinking that they are simply moody and unpredictable.

Criteria for Diagnosing ADHD in Kids

It is important to keep in mind that not every kid who is hyperactive, overly impulsive, or inattentive, is suffering from ADHD. Sometimes, kids simply blurt out things that they didn't mean to say in the first place. Likewise, they are sometimes forgetful and disorganized and even jump from one unfinished task to another. Exhibiting such behaviors doesn't necessarily mean that they have ADHD. Every kid shows these symptoms at some point in their lives. Diagnosing ADHD requires that these symptoms must have been demonstrated over a long time. The behaviors ought to have appeared early in a kids' life (before the age of 7 years), and must have been exhibited for more than 6 months. The behaviors must also have caused a notable handicap in more than two areas of a kid's life, such as in the learning environment and in social settings.

If a kid exhibits some ADHD-related symptoms, yet his/her schoolwork or social interactions are not affected, it would be wrong to diagnose that kid as having ADHD. Besides this, a kid who seems to be overly hyperactive in class, yet functions well elsewhere, can't receive an ADHD diagnosis. To establish whether kids have ADHD, specialists often ask several critical questions; are the behaviors exhibited by a kid excessive? Are they pervasive and long-term? Do they occur in only one specific place or in several settings? In addition, specialists also need to establish whether the behaviors in question occur more frequently in a kid than in other children of the same age. This will help assess whether the behaviors are a continuous problem or simply responses to temporary solutions.

When diagnosing ADHD in kids, their behavioral pattern is typically compared to a specified set of criteria. ADHD-related characteristics are thereafter listed in the DSM-IV-TR (Diagnostic and Statistical Manual of Mental Disorders). This is a manual published by the American Psychiatric Association to provide a common language and standardized criteria for classifying mental disorders.

Diagnosing ADHD in Kids

Most parents notice signs of hyperactivity, impulsivity, and inattention in their kids before they start schooling. Your preschool kid could have ADHD if he/she loses interest when playing games or watching TV, or even seemingly randomly lose control.

Kids have different personalities, energy levels, and temperaments. They also mature at different rates. Therefore it is advisable to get a behavioral expert's opinion to determine the behavior that is appropriate for your kids at their age. If you suspect that your child has ADHD, you can ask a child psychologist or psychiatrist to either confirm or dispel your fears. Keep in mind that kids often exhibit unusually exuberant and immature behavior and, therefore, you shouldn't hastily conclude that yours has ADHD without having him/her diagnosed by a specialist.

In most cases, ADHD in kids is usually suspected by parents but, nonetheless, remains ignored until they start having problems in school or in their social interactions. Given the fact that the condition tends to mostly affect kids' functioning at school, it is common for teachers to be the first ones to suspect its presence. Once teachers recognize that a kid in their class exhibits prolonged inattentiveness or hyperactivity, it is advisable that they point it out to parents so that ADHD diagnosis and subsequent treatment is undertaken. Since teachers spend time with lots of kids, it is easy for them to know how "normal" kids behave within the class environment. They similarly know how "abnormal" kids behave. Therefore, they are in the best position to inform you whether your kid exhibits prolonged strange behavior in class.

A kid can only be diagnosed with ADHD if he/she exhibits more than six of the nine ADHD symptoms. Similarly, the symptoms must have been observed for more than six months and in more than two settings. It must also be proved that the symptoms are adversely affecting the behavior of that kid. Some of these symptoms must also have been observed before the age of 12.

Who Should Diagnose ADHD in Kids?

Many parents do not know who they should turn to once they suspect ADHD in the kids. Ideally, ADHD diagnosis should be made by child psychologists/psychiatrists, behavioral neurologists, or behavioral/development pediatricians. Clinical social workers can also diagnose ADHD, especially those who have handled similar cases in the past.

Several specialists are qualified to both diagnose and treat the symptoms of ADHD. These specialists can undertake the assessment themselves, or they can serve family members with questionnaires to determine the kids' behavior. Regardless of a specialists' area of expertise, his/her first task should be gathering information that will help rule out various other possible reasons for the kids' behavior.

Possible causes of ADHD-like behavior among kids may include:

- sudden changes in their lives such as their parents' divorce
- unnoticed disorders, such as seizures, including temporal lobe or petit mal seizures
- mental disorders that affect the brain functionality of kids

- middle ear infection, which leads to intermittent hearing problems

- anxiety or depression

- underachievement caused by common learning disabilities

The above mentioned are some of the ADHD-like symptoms that lead parents to suspect that their kids could be suffering from the behavioral disorder. When diagnosing ADHD, these symptoms ought to be ruled out for the diagnosis to be accurate. Ruling out such symptoms when diagnosing ADHD may involve going through a kid's medical and school records. Once it is determined that the kid isn't suffering from any of these conditions, specialists should gather information pertaining to a child's ongoing behavior. This will help them compare their behavior with diagnostic criteria and symptoms that are listed in the DSM-IV-TR. Talking to the child or even observing them in their learning environment and other social settings can go a long way in helping specialists gauge their ongoing behavior.

Diagnosing ADHD in kids should also involve asking teachers about their observations pertaining to the young ones' behavior. These observations should be noted down on standard evaluation forms, which are typically referred to as behavior rating scales. These scales help compare a kid's behavior with that of other children of the same age. Even though rating scales are sometimes overly subjective, they give teachers a valid and reliable measure for determining the long-term behavior of kids under their care.

During diagnosis, specialists can contact anyone who knows the affected kids well, including family members, coaches, and babysitters. Such individuals may be asked to describe the kids' behavior in various situations. In addition, they might also be required to fill out questionnaires or rating scales so that the specialists can determine how frequent and severe the behaviors are.

When diagnosing ADHD among children, their mental health and social adjustment are the main pillars of the assessment. Besides this, learning achievement and intelligence tests may also be given to determine whether the kids have a learning difficulty.

When looking at the results of various information sources, specialists often pay more attention to the kids' behavior in situations that demand a high degree of self-control. This may include noisy and unstructured circumstances, such as parties and activities that require sustained mental effort; examples can be playing board games or working out mathematical problems.

During ADHD diagnosis, kids' behavior and interaction during free play or when they are given individual attention is usually given less importance. In such circumstances, most children who have ADHD tend to control their behavior and even perform better than when they are in restrictive situations.

After the behavior of kids, who are suspected of having ADHD, has been evaluated over time, specialists often put together a profile that summarizes the observations made over the course of the evaluation. This profile helps the specialists pinpoint ADHD-like behaviors, which are listed in the most recent DSM (Diagnostic and Statistical Manual). A profile similarly helps specialists to determine how frequently these behaviors are exhibited by a kid, whether or not they are periodic in nature, and how long the behaviors are exhibited in each instance. If a kid has any other problems that are related to ADHD, they will also be captured in the profile. Ultimately, the profile will help a specialist determine whether a kid's hyperactivity-impulsivity, inattention, or both, is significant and longstanding. If so, it can be correctly concluded that the kid has ADHD.

A correct diagnosis of ADHD will go a long way in resolving the confusion surrounding a kid's learning problems. It similarly provides the correct information as to what exactly is "wrong" with a kid, and what needs to be done to mitigate the symptoms of the disorder. Thereafter, therapy and medication can be recommended. The kid's family members will also be given educational material about managing ADHD.

Which Other Disorders Accompany ADHD Among Kids?

Learning Disabilities

A significant number of kids with ADHD (30-40%) tend to have specific learning disabilities. In pre-school kids, these learning disabilities are manifested by difficulties in understanding certain words or sounds, and even difficulties in expressing oneself clearly. In school-going children, ADHD-related learning difficulties are typically manifested by spelling or reading disabilities, arithmetic disorders, and writing disorders. Dyslexia, a common type of reading disorder is also quite widespread among children who have ADHD. Even though reading disabilities are common with kids who have ADHD, up to 8% of elementary school kids experience reading difficulties at some point. However, this shouldn't suggest that they also have ADHD.

Tourette Syndrome

An insignificant percentage of kids with ADHD also have Tourette Syndrome. This neurological disorder is characterized by repetitive mannerisms and nervous tics. This may include facial twitches, grimacing, and eye blinks. Others have the tendency to frequently clear their throats, sniff, bark out words, or snort. Behaviors that are related to Tourette Syndrome can easily be treated using medication. Even though very few kids are affected by this disorder, a significant number of those who have it also have ADHD.

Oppositional Defiant Disorder

Up to 50% of kids with ADHD also have oppositional defiant disorder (ODD). This disorder is characterized by non-compliant, defiant, stubborn, and sometimes belligerent behavior among kids. Children who suffer from this disorder tend to experience incessant outbursts of temper and are generally disobedient and argumentative. ODD affects children suffering from hyperactive-impulsivity, inattentive, and combined ADHD types.

Conduct Disorder

Between 20 to 40% of children with ADHD end up developing conduct disorder (CD). This disorder is basically a more serious and complex form of antisocial behavior. Children who have the disorder tend to have antisocial mannerisms such as lying, stealing, bullying others, or fighting. This puts them at risk of falling foul with the law or being aggressive towards everyone around them. As they get older, children who have conduct disorder are at a great risk of drug and substance use.

Anxiety and Depression

Some kids who have ADHD struggle with co-occurring depression and anxiety. Such kids will be in a better position to handle some of the symptoms that accompany ADHD if the anxiety and depression is detected early and treated. Likewise, if ADHD is effectively treated, depression and anxiety among kids is also likely to reduce significantly. This makes it easier for them to handle academic tasks and any other duties that they are asked to perform.

Bipolar Disorder

It is difficult to distinguish between ADHD and bipolar disorder among kids since both conditions have similar symptoms. In its purest form, bipolar disorder is typified by mood swings between periods of extreme highs and lows. Nonetheless, bipolar in children is often a somewhat chronic mood deregulation characterized by a mix of elation, irritability, and depression. Besides this, there are certain symptoms that are present in kids suffering from both bipolar disorder and ADHD, including a decreased need for sleep and high energy levels. Of the main symptoms that are present in kids with bipolar disorder from those with ADHD, grandiosity and elated mood are the distinguishing characteristics.

Chapter 3: Attention Deficit Hyperactivity Disorder in Adults

ADHD among children is so publicized to the extent that not many people know that the disorder also affects adults. What many people don't know is the fact that all kids who have ADHD will still have it in their adult years. Research indicates that up to 70% of children who have ADHD will exhibit symptoms of the disorder during their adult years.

The first study conducted on grown-ups who had never been diagnosed with ADHD during their childhood but showed symptoms of the disorder as adults, was conducted by David Wood, Paul Wender, and Frederick Reimherr. The symptomatic adults were diagnosed with ADHD retrospectively after the researchers interviewed their parents. Ultimately, the trio came up with the Utah criteria, which is a clinical framework for diagnosing adults with ADHD. Generally, the diagnosis of adult ADHD involves evaluating the history of patients, and assessing it against current ADHD-like behaviors. At the moment, there are other diagnostic evaluations for determining the presence of adult ADHD. These include the use of the widely-popular Conners Comprehensive Behavior Rating Scale (Conners CBRS) and the Brown ADD Scales.

It's extremely common for adults who have ADHD to not realize that they have the disorder in the fact place. In cases whereby the disorder was diagnosed and treated in childhood, most adults end up believing that it was fully mitigated and, therefore, it doesn't affect them in adulthood. Whichever the case, adults who have ADHD often feel it is just impossible for them to get organized or even stick to one job for a substantial period. Others even find it difficult to stick to schedules or even keep an appointment. Everyday tasks such as waking up on time, getting to work early, or staying productive at work can be significant challenges to adults who have ADHD.

Symptoms of Adult ADHD

ADHD in adults manifests itself in various ways. Just like with children, adult ADHD can be in the form of hyperactivity and impulsivity, inattention, or a combination of the two. It should be noted that while it isn't difficult to spot ADHD in children, it is hard to in adults. This is attributed to the fact that adults tend to have subtle symptoms, which are hard to spot. This explains why, in most cases, adults struggle with the disorder without knowing that they have it. They fail to recognize that most of the problems that they face in their lives, including staying organized or arriving for meetings on time, relate to ADHD.

Hyperactivity-Impulsivity Symptoms in Adults

If you have the tendency of fidgeting, squirming in your seat, tapping your hands and feet, you probably have adult ADHD. Those who leave their seats even when they are required to remain seated, especially within the workplace setting, could also have ADHD. The disorder is also manifested in instances when you find yourself running where it is inappropriate, or you find it difficult to take part in leisure activities quietly and without feeling restless.

Adults who suffer from the hypersensitive-impulsive type of ADHD sometimes act as if they are "on the go" or they are being driven by an underlying force. This makes it difficult for them to remain still for extended periods of time, such as when in meetings and restaurants. The tendency to talk excessively while often blurting out answers even before questions have been fully asked could be a sign that an adult it battling with hypersensitive-impulsive ADHD. Such individuals tend to complete other people's sentences, and find it hard to wait for their turn when carrying out conversations. They also tend to intrude into activities and take over from others without seeking permission.

Inattentive ADHD Symptoms in Adults

Adults who find it hard to organize tasks and activities, manage time, and meet deadlines, may also have inattentive ADHD. Besides this, the tendency to avoid, dislike, or show reluctance towards participation in tasks that require concerted or sustained mental effort, points towards inattentive ADHD. This form of ADHD is also manifested in adults who often lose items such as work tools, keys, wallet, important documents, mobile phones, and eyeglasses, and those who easily get distracted when undertaking important things by unrelated thoughts. Forgetfulness in daily tasks such as running errands, paying bills, and returning calls also is a manifestation of inattentive ADHD.

Some adults who suffer from inattentive ADHD may seem not to be carefully listening even when they are spoken to directly. Their minds may be elsewhere even in instances where there seems to be no obvious distraction. Besides this, they often fail to follow through any instructions given to them or duties that they are allocated. Even in instances when they start tasks, they will lose focus quickly or easily get sidetracked.

The Appearance of ADHD Symptoms Amongst Adults

Generally, ADHD among adults appears in different settings. Adults can get affected by ADHD at home, at work, in social situations, or anywhere else. For a positive diagnosis of the behavioral disorder to be made, the aforementioned symptoms ought to be present in more than one setting. Besides this, the symptoms ought to occur more often. ADHD may also appear differently among adults. There must also be evidence that the ADHD symptoms that an adult portrayed interfered with his/her work, academic, and social functions. The symptoms should also not be due to a different mental or behavioral disorder.

Since the condition is a lifelong disorder, which is less noticeable in adults than in kids, many people tend to think that it is less serious during adulthood. What you may not know is the fact that during adulthood, you are vested with more responsibilities and, therefore, any mistake that you make as a result of ADHD is likely to have greater consequences to you and others. For this reason, diagnosing and treating ADHD in adults is just as important as diagnosing and treating it in children.

Diagnosing ADHD in Adults

It isn't easy to diagnose ADHD in adults. Whenever children get diagnosed with ADHD, in most cases parents tend to remember that they may have had the same symptoms during their childhood. This makes them understand some of the behaviors and traits such as restlessness, impulsivity, and distractibility, which are giving their kids problems. Likewise, some adults often discover that they have ADHD after they seek professional help for mental disorders such as anxiety or depression, only to discover that the root of their emotional disorder is ADHD.

For adults to be diagnosed with ADHD, they must have ADHD-like symptoms that started in childhood. Those symptoms must be persistent and current. The accuracy of ADHD diagnosis in adults is important and, therefore, a diagnosis should only be made by a specialist who has specialized in the field of attention dysfunction. For a diagnosis to be accurate, the behavioral history of patients since childhood needs to be evaluated. In addition, interviews with patients' life partner, parents, family members or close associates will be required. Psychological tests and physical examinations can also be undertaken to establish whether one's condition is related to other conditions such as anxiety, learning disabilities, or affective disorders.

To diagnose ADHD in older teens and adults, they must have demonstrated the symptoms of different ADHD types in multiple settings. For instance, if an adult fails to hold down one job for a considerable period, a diagnosis could help unravel whether ADHD is the underlying cause behind this situation. Just like it is the case when diagnosing ADHD in kids, the symptoms must have been observed for a considerable period, and in different settings.

Adults who have struggled with ADHD unknowingly for years often have a sense of relief after a correct diagnosis of the disorder has been made. Typically, individuals who have unknowingly suffered from ADHD bring many negative perceptions about themselves into adulthood due to the effect that the condition has had on them. Once past and present behaviors that are related to ADHD have been brought into perspective, it is easy for one to face them head-on. This could perhaps explain why ADHD treatment in adults mostly entails psychotherapy since it helps them cope with whatever anger they might feel owing to the failure to diagnose the condition during their childhood or younger years.

Couples with ADHD
If an adult has ADHD, it is obvious that the first person who will be affected is his/her spouse/partner Needless to say, the disorder can put an end to even the closest of relationships. Symptoms such as procrastination, distraction, and

impulsivity, can stir feelings such as hunger and frustration, besides hurting the other party's feelings. When such a situation occurs in both adults with ADHD and their partners can be affected and, consequently, drift apart. Nevertheless, the relationship can still thrive even one partner has ADHD. Proper treatment and coping tactics can help couples ward off the devastating effects of ADHD.

Couples' Expectation Guide on ADHD Marriage

Distraction

Distraction is among the commonest ADHD symptoms. If one of the couple has ADHD, chances are high that most times, he/she won't seem to listen whenever the other speaks to them. Such individuals may also constantly fail to follow through on any promises made to their partners. Love still exists, but they tend to get distracted by their phones, the TV, or, sometimes, just their own thoughts.

How to Deal With Distraction

The fact that one partner easily gets distracted, or tends to wander off whenever a discussion is being held, doesn't mean that he/she no longer cares about the other. Once this symptom is noticed over a prolonged period and in different settings, a diagnosis should be considered as soon as possible. Being open, in a calm manner, about feelings of how this makes the other feel is equally important. Bottling up feelings, anger, and emotion can lead to spousal resentment.

If the constant distraction is causing conversations to be a real problem, finding the most appropriate time when they get least distracted is a good idea. Sometimes, it helps to touch their arms when talking to them so that they notice the other's presence. This will make it hard for them to drift away. To connect with an ADHD partner during conversations, establish what makes them drift away. Thereafter, avoid situations that make them get distracted. In addition, keep conversations brief because it will be harder for them to become uninterested and distracted.

Hyper-focus

This is the opposite of distraction, and another symptom of ADHD. ADHD adults who experience hyperfocus tend to get so engrossed in an activity that it makes it hard to shift their attention away. Hyperfocus can be advantageous, especially in cases where it enhances an individual's productivity. Nonetheless, it can also be disastrous if left unchecked. Loved ones, in particular, are the ones who are likely to bear the brunt of hyperfocus because they might feel less important, simply because something that doesn't seem to be important has taken away their loved ones' attention.

Dealing With Hyperfocus

If a spouse is prone to spells of hyperfocus when undertaking certain activities, such as creating puzzles, it's best for the other to engage them elsewhere. Scheduling such activities far away from mealtimes or moments when partners need to interact with each other will help. Those who portray symptoms of hyperfocus can set alarms to track time that they spent on one activity. This will help them move to equally important activities when they realize that they are hyper-focused. Partners shouldn't take it personally if their spouses have the habit of being hyper-focused on other activities.

Forgetfulness

It's often the case that one partner thinks the other is being forgetful for the sake of it. The truth of the matter is that he/she could be battling with ADHD unknowingly. Without a diagnosis, a level of distrust could sink in towards the ADHD partner even with basic tasks. For the partner with ADHD and they don't realize this to be the case, they may end up feeling like a failure. Ultimately, anger will build up on both sides.

Forgetfulness Strategies

Forgetfulness isn't a character flaw like many people have been led to believe. If one partner has the tendency of forgetting even basic things, the other can make an effort to seek a diagnosis. Avoid labeling this ADHD symptom as being uncaring or being rude. Also, giving the ADHD partner lengthy lectures will only make him/her fall deeper into self-pity and resentment, towards the other. Focusing on working with your spouse to help him/her remember tasks that they are to undertake will help. A daily planner or task reminders on their phones will also come in handy.

Disorganization

ADHD adults are likely to have the disorganization trait. Such individuals are likely to leave their jobs unfinished or even skip their chores altogether, lose important documents, car keys, and phones. Disorganization not only leads to stress but also wastage. Trying to give a lecture to an adult with ADHD who is disorganized can leave him/her feeling controlled.

How to Cope With Disorganization

Whenever a spouse is disorganized, the other should try to sit him/her down and talk to them calmly. One maybe disorganized when undertaking some roles but can be more organized in others. Understanding each other's strengths when undertaking tasks will go a long way in preventing chore wars. Besides this, respecting the ADHD partner's habit of keeping items in certain spots might be difficult but will be rewarding. In as much that the placement of the items in those spots might look clumsy; it could be their way of keeping things organized.

Impulsivity

Adults who have the hyperactive form of ADHD tend to make impulsive decisions. They will act without thinking. In marriages, the main problem that hyperactive ADHD couples may experience is impulsive spending. One may have the habit of buying things out-of-the-blue without consulting the other, or considering the family unit's financial situation. Some of the items might even be irrelevant or might be viewed as being extravagant and inconsiderate. Either way, the underlying cause of the impulsivity could be ADHD. If a partner has risqué sexual habits, drives dangerously, or often blurts out unsuitable comments in social occasions, he/she could be driven by impulsivity.

Handling Impulsivity

Managing impulsivity in a marriage setting entails a lot of self-control, which can actually be learned. Aiding a partner to develop self-control in all situations can be done through role-playing, so that they learn how to act in different situations. If they have the habit of overspending on their credit cards, teaching them how to write shopping lists and also why they should leave their credit cards at home when going shopping will help. The most crucial thing about managing impulsivity is cutting out temptation. If the impulsive behaviors get out of hand, therapy definitely needs to be sought.

Procrastination

Everyone has a habit of putting off tasks that appear boring or difficult. In a marriage setting, this habit can be detrimental because relationships involve playing differing roles in the household and relationship. An ADHD adult who has the habit of procrastinating may not know how to undertake tasks, or they might feel overwhelmed. They only tend to get started when deadlines are on the horizon. This is a recipe for chaotic lifestyles, which may ultimately cause couples to drift apart.

Avoiding Procrastination

Most adults who tend to push forward their roles have the inattention type of ADHD. They feel overwhelmed by tasks that often appear too big to handle. Rather than letting them struggle with such tasks, the other partner can work with them to break the project into smaller tasks that are easy to tackle. Sharing duties within the task will give the other partner some company and support since it will make them tail off. ADHD adults shouldn't look at procrastination as a defect but rather as a trait that is manageable.

Mood Swings

Individuals who have ADHD often exhibit erratic behavior, which is characterized by a shift between spells of happiness and moodiness. They also have difficulty when it comes to controlling their emotions; they might want to lash out in anger when their moods set in simply because they feel anxious or frustrated. If this is the case and the ADHD us undiagnosed their behavior might compromise the relationship.

Managing Mood Swings

Normally, a partner's mood swings are caused by events happening around them. Therefore, lifestyle changes can go a long way in alleviating the erratic moods. A healthy diet, regular exercise, and ample sleep will go a long way in preventing the mood swings. Keep in mind that a spouse's moods swings can only be eased is he/she learns how to control their impulses. For the other partner, avoid topics and conversations that may lead to overreactions and flare-ups. In as much as their situation should be empathized with, an explanation as to their mood swings affect the other is important. With time, they will learn how to control their emotions.

ADHD And Intimacy

Couples who have ADHD often have problems as far as communication and intimacy are concerned. If you have ADHD, you may experience trouble paying attention to your partner. Your mind might wander even during the most intimate moments with your spouse. This will seem normal to you but nonetheless, your partner is likely to see it as lack of interest. With time, a lack of attention may breed resentment, which in turn causes spouses to drift apart. ADHD adults are also likely to be drawn to risky sexual behaviors such as unprotected sexual encounters. ADHD often lowers the level of neurotransmitters, thus putting you at risk of being impulsive and taking risks.

Married couples who have ADHD are bound to realize that the condition often affects their relationship in many ways. Distractibility and inattention, which are among the main ADHD symptoms, often subverts eroticism and romance. However, this doesn't mean that ADHD and intimacy cannot coexist. Couples should find a way of keeping their intimacy intact even when one of them has ADHD.

Spouses with ADHD must find a way of rebalancing their relationship. Similarly should work towards letting go of any resentment that might have cropped up as a result of the condition. Talking to a therapist can go a long way in helping rekindle the long-lost intimacy. ADHD couples who have kids should learn to share responsibilities pertaining to childcare, money and organization. Ultimately, their romance will be reawakened.

It is generally advisable for couples to address the big challenges that face their relationship while finding new ways of learning communication skills. This will not only bridge their differences but also minimize whatever resentment that might have cropped up. In this regard, couples need to hone their speaking and listening skills while discussing their challenges without being aggressive or listening defensively. This will help them maintain or discover their affection towards each other. When dealing with ADHD as a couple, it is always good to let the partner know how one feels.

ADHD at the Workplace

There are certain attributes that employers often look out for before hiring staff. These include excellent focus, speed, organization, an ability to meet deadlines, and attention to detail. If you have ADHD, meeting such requirements can be quite a challenge. Even when you are on the job, excelling in your roles ends up being a tall order, thus making it difficult for you to keep the job, let alone getting promoted. This shouldn't mean that you can't excel in a career if you have ADHD. Sometimes, the disorder can be an asset to you and your workmates.

How ADHD Affects Employment

Up to 9 million adults in the U.S. have ADHD. This represents a significant percentage of the American workforce. Studies have shown that adults with ADHD often struggle at work. A national survey indicated that only 50% of adults who have ADHD are able to maintain a full-time job. On the flipside, 72%

of adults without ADHD can hold down a full-time job. Whenever ADHD adults land a job, they tend to earn slightly less than their colleagues who do not have the disorder.

The extent to which the disorder affects your employment outlook depends on its severity. While some individuals may only have problems when it comes to staying on one task, others find it hard to work all day without getting into a blow-up with their co-workers or superiors. Those who are severely affected by ADHD may end up moving from one job to another. In extreme cases, they even end up seeking disability benefits.

Generally, this behavioral disorder affects job performance in various ways. If you cannot sit still during meetings or you have difficulties staying focused and organized, it will be hard for you to stay on one job for a substantial amount of time. Typically, individuals battling with ADHD have trouble with working memory, attention, verbal fluency, and mental processing. These qualities are generally referred to as executive-function abilities, and they come in handy at the workplace. Within the work environment, it is easy for you to get depressed or have low self-esteem if you have difficulties completing your tasks within schedules or beating simple deadlines. This may make your situation even worse.

How ADHD Adults Can Succeed at Work

Adults who lack the ability to concentrate or are restless, often haven't been diagnosed with ADHD. If you experience any ADHD-related symptoms, it is advisable that you have the disorder diagnosed and managed accordingly. Once medication and therapy starts you will find it easier to manage your daily roles and even succeed in your career and social life. ADHD adults are often advised to work with career counselors when embarking on a job search. This goes a long way in helping them land jobs that match their abilities, needs, and interests. Depending on your ADHD, you may want to find employment in either a fast-paced environment, or a less rigid one.

Once you have landed a job, there are certain strategies that can help you manage your ADHD. Find peace in whatever work environment you find yourself in. Ask to be allocated a quiet working space where it won't be easy for you to get distracted. If you have trouble organizing your tasks and schedule, work with a colleague or superior who is well-organized so that you are guided through projects. Besides this, always maintain a daily planner with a to-do list and a calendar. Have electronic reminders about due dates and meetings to keep you updated with what you are supposed to do.

To keep your memory fresh, always take notes during meetings and also when making work-related phone calls. Add these notes to your diary and to-do lists. You should also schedule interruptions by setting aside specific periods for answering your calls or emails. This will ensure that your schedule and more important responsibilities are not interrupted. When undertaking tasks, you should set realistic goals for yourself while bearing in mind that you have ADHD. Break up every workday into a series of assignments and, thereafter, attempt to tackle each small assignment one at a time. In this regard, have a timer that will notify you when to move to the next task.

To effectively manage ADHD at work, it is advisable that you always reward yourself after completing tasks. Taking a break or even stepping out of the office for a break is a worthy reward. For bigger accomplishments, you should even consider buying yourself something that you've always wanted. To avoid a breakdown that typifies ADHD symptoms, you should be ready to delegate smaller tasks so that you can focus on more important ones. This will also prevent loss of focus as a result of distractions. What's more, you should always make it a habit to relax. This will help ramp up our energy levels, thus boosting your concentration.

How ADHD Can be Beneficial At Work

ADHD is categorized as a disability under the Americans with Disabilities Act. Employers are required to accommodate the needs of employees who have ADHD without discriminating against them. You need to be bold enough to inform your employer that you have ADHD. Unbeknown to many people, ADHD can be used to a positive effect at work. The impulsiveness, desire to try out new things, and restlessness can be great assets if harnessed properly. These ADHD symptoms particularly come in handy if you run your own business. The trick lies in finding a career that suits you and uses your boundless energy, creativity, and other strengths to your benefit.

With necessary support, adults who have ADHD can be productive members of the workplace. For instance, an ADHD symptom such as hyperfocus ought to be harnessed so that these individuals are allowed to work on projects that they are most interested in. They are likely to focus intensely on such projects, something that will ultimately result in positive results.

Hyperfocus is advantageous owing to the fact that it can help employees to channel their attention and energy into whatever projects that they handle. The ability to focus for hours on end particularly comes in handy in careers such as science, writing, and art. ADHD adults are generally advised not to wallow in their condition. Instead, they should be proud of the out-of-the-box thinking, passion, and drive that it brings. Looking at the condition in a positive light will go a long way in helping them manage it.

The lack of awareness about ADHD means that many adult patients end up being misunderstood or misinterpreted at their workplaces due to their inconsistency. As a result, many of them struggle to hold down one job for a considerable period. Proper diagnosis and management of the condition can go a long way in enabling ADHD adults to make the most of their talents.

Chapter 4: Medical and Treatment Guidance for ADHD

Medication for ADHD Types

The three types of ADHD exhibit varying symptoms and, as a result, they should be treated differently. Besides differences in medications used, the kind of therapy that ought to be offered for the three ADHD types also varies. In addition, treatment for kids with ADHD varies from treatment offered to adults.

Medication for Hypersensitive-Impulsive ADHD Type

Individuals who have this type of ADHD often exhibit strong emotional reaction towards things and circumstances that "normal" people take in their stride. The heightened and over-the-top reactions are typically emotional in nature, and may arise from rather negative or positive situations. It isn't unusual for individuals who have hypersensitive-impulsive ADHD to be physically sensitive to common senses such as light, sound, and touch. More than 50% of individuals with this ADHD type have difficulties with emotional regulation and, therefore, they experience symptoms such as temper outbursts, impulsivity, mood fluctuations, and low tolerance levels.

Antidepressants are the most widely-used medicines as far as the treatment of hypersensitive-impulsive ADHD is concerned. Common antidepressants used to treat this disorder include bupropion, desipramine, imipramine, and nortriptyline. Each of these medicines has its side effects, but the severity of the symptoms depends on the dosage with which the medicines are administered. Bupropion may cause headaches in rare cases. It also increases the risk of seizures and, therefore, an individual's medical history ought to be evaluated before the drug is administered. Desipramine isn't recommended for use among children with hypersensitive-impulsive ADHD. The drug is associated with some rare cases of heart ailments. Imipramine may cause several side effects, including fatigue, anxiety, stomach upsets, increased risk of arrhythmias, elevated heartbeat, and dry mouth. These side effects may also be present in individuals with hypersensitive-impulsive ADHD who are treated with nortriptyline.

Generally, antidepressants are considered to be safe, especially if the dosage is administered by a professional. Rarely do serious problems arise after the drugs have been administered. Besides this, not all hypersensitive-impulsive patients will exhibit the aforementioned side effects once these drugs have been administered.

Medication for Inattentive ADHD

Individuals suffering from inattentive ADHD often have problems staying alert over longer periods. In most cases, stimulant medication is recommended to enable their brains to send and receive signals, thus enabling them to pay attention for longer periods, and also to think more clearly. The most common medications used to manage inattentive ADHD include amphetamine-based and methylphenidate-based medicines. Once inattentive ADHD has been diagnosed, the medical practitioner will recommend a low dose of the aforementioned medicines to see whether your symptoms will be controlled. If it doesn't, the dose may be slowly increased.

Most medicines used to treat inattentive ADHD come in short-term and long-term acting forms. The former typically wear off in around 4 hours. Therefore, you are required to take them once or twice daily. On the other hand, long-acting stimulants wear off after 8-12 hours. You are only required to take these once a day. For inattentive ADHD treatment, to achieve the most suitable outcome, it is advisable that you talk with your doctor so that you decide on the medication that works best for you. In this regard, you should consider your daily routine so that you figure out the best schedule for taking your medication.

ADHD patients should avoid taking stimulants if they have serious health disorders such as glaucoma, a history of substance and alcohol abuse, and heart disease. If you are taking an antidepressant while under treatment for inattentive ADHD, you should consult your doctor before embarking on stimulant medication. You also need to keep in mind that stimulants cause side effects, such as mouth dryness, headaches, insomnia, and loss of appetite. If you also take medication via patches on your skin, the skin color in those specific areas is likely to change. You shouldn't be worried about the side effects of stimulant medication because, in most cases, they disappear on their own within a few days or weeks of commencing medication. If you feel that the side effects are a bother, consult your doctor so that a different drug is prescribed to you, or the dosage is changed.

Non-Stimulant Medication for ADHD

Non-stimulant medication can also be used to treat ADHD. This route is normally taken when treating combined type ADHD. In addition, non-stimulant medication can be used on individuals who experience drastic side effects to stimulant medication. Anti-stimulants, such as atomoxetine are administered to raise chemical levels in the brains of ADHD patients, helping to control their behavior. These usually take several weeks to start working and if they are administered to you, you may experience side effects such as heartburn, constipation, and diminished sex drive; all of which will wear off in time. In case you cannot take other ADHD medication, your doctor may prescribe either clonidine or guanfacine, which are blood pressure drugs that can help you manage ADHD symptoms such as hyperactivity and impulsivity.

Treatment in Kids

To treat ADHD among kids effectively, families need to work with the healthcare professional who diagnosed the disorder in the first place. According to the Multimodal Treatment Study of Children with Attention Deficit Hyperactivity Disorder (MTA), one intervention cannot work in isolation as far as the treatment of ADHD is concerned. Medical management ought to be blended with behavioral treatment and routine community care for optimal outcomes to be attained.

Most kids who are diagnosed with this behavioral disorder are given medication. Stimulants and methylphenidates are the most common medications used. It is always advisable that children only be introduced to medication after behavioral therapy has been undertaken. Keep in mind that, when it comes to ADHD, no individual treatment strategy works for every child. Besides this, children sometimes have adverse side effects when subjected to a particular medication. In such situations, that particular treatment will be rendered unacceptable.

Medical Interventions for ADHD Kids

For years, various medicines have been used in the treatment of ADHD among kids. Generally, these medications only treat symptoms of the disorder. Stimulants have for long been regarded as the most effective medication as far as managing the symptoms of ADHD is concerned. Stimulants are often used to lower kids' impulsivity and hyperactivity thus improving their ability to focus on one activity at a time. This allows them to work and even learn new skills. Amphetamines are approved for use on ADHD children who are between the ages of 3 and 5. On the other hand, methylphenidates are typically used to treat the symptoms of ADHD among kids who are older than. Some of the amphetamines that are prescribed for kids with ADHD are meant to improve their physical coordination. The prescribing physician and the diagnosing specialist ought to work together to determine the right medication and dosage for each individual case.

Stimulants that are used to remedy ADHD among children are generally considered to be quite safe since they do not make the kids feel "high." Nevertheless, some kids may still feel funny or slightly different after using this medication. Stimulants used to treat ADHD among kids do not lead to dependence or drug abuse.

A paltry percentage of kids with ADHD are not helped by stimulant medication. Other medications can also be prescribed if ADHD occurs alongside another disorder. This includes antidepressants, which are typically administered to reduce anxiety or depression.

When using medicines as part of the interventions against ADHD symptoms, it is important to take note of a number of facts. Medications improve kids' focus thus helping them improve in school and in their overall social interactions. In addition, more than 80% of kids who need medication to mitigate the symptoms of ADHD will still need it when they enter their teenage years. 50% of them will need medication as adults.

Medication and behavioral therapy go a long way in mitigating ADHD among kids. Nevertheless, family members play the most crucial part. For this reason, both ADHD kids and their family members need special help since it will help them develop strategies for managing behavior patterns. Mental health professionals may be needed to counsel both the kids and their families in view of helping them develop new attitudes, skills, and ways of relating with each other. When counseling children who have ADHD, therapists should help them learn ways of feeling better about themselves. They should also help the kids identify and work on their strengths besides learning how to cope with problems that they face in their lives. In addition, they should also be taught how to manage their attention and aggression.

Every member of the family will be affected if a child has ADHD. Consequently, the entire family will need help so that everyone learns how to cope with the condition. Since kids with ADHD often have disruptive behaviors, therapists should focus on finding ways of handling such behaviors. This may entail teaching parents and other family members some techniques for coping with the behaviors and how to improve them.

Psychotherapy doesn't address the underlying causes or symptoms of ADHD. It basically entails the kids and their families talking to the therapist about upsetting feelings and thoughts. This helps them explore self-defeating behavioral patterns besides learning alternative ways of handling their emotions. As family members and parents talk to therapists, they will be able to understand how to deal with the disorder in a better way.

Behavioral therapists help ADHD kids and their families to develop ways of handling immediate issues that may arise. Rather than helping the kids understand their feelings and actions, behavioral therapy helps them change their thinking and, consequently, leads to changes in their behavior. This kind of support is akin to practical assistance, which helps them become more organized when undertaking their tasks, as well as helping them deal with emotionally-charged events.

Social-skills training can help children who have ADHD to learn new behaviors. This basically involves therapists discussing with the kids and their families appropriate behaviors that help build and maintain social relationships, such as waiting for a turn, responding to teasing, and asking for help. For instance, the kids might be taught how to read people's facial expressions and voice tones, so that they learn how to respond appropriately.

Support groups can be used to help parents connect with other parents whose kids are suffering from ADHD. Support groups members can meet on a regular basis and listen to behavioral experts so that they learn how best to deal with their kids' situation. Support groups similarly enable parents to share their successes and failures as far as managing their ADHD is concerned. They can also obtain referrals to experts and pertinent information in dealing with ADHD.

Parental skills training is offered either in special classes or by behavioral therapists to parents, with the objective of giving them techniques for managing their kids' behavior. The most common technique is rewarding good behavior and isolating them when they misbehave. This system of rewards and sanctions is an effective way of modifying a kid's behavior. When kids are rewarded for good behavior or completing tasks, they identify desirable behaviors that they should uphold, and undesirable behaviors to avoid. Over time, such techniques help ADHD kids to learn how to control their behavior and thus choose those ones that are desirable. When handling their ADHD kids, parents also need to learn ways of structuring situations in a manner that allows their kids to succeed. This includes allowing them to interact with several playmates at a time. Their children won't be overstimulated to be hyperactive or impulsive, or inattentive in such cases. If your kid has difficulties completing tasks, you can help them learn to do so by dividing large tasks into smaller bits. The kid should be praised and rewarded as he/she completes the smaller tasks.

Parents should also learn how to use stress management techniques such as relaxation methods, exercise, and meditation. This will increase their tolerance for frustration thus enabling them to respond more calmly to their kid's behavior.

Strategies for Family with ADHD

Medication and behavioral therapy go a long way in mitigating ADHD among kids. Nevertheless, family members play the most crucial part. For this reason, both ADHD kids and their family members need special help, for it will help them develop strategies for managing behavior patterns. Mental health professionals may be needed to counsel both the kids and their families in view of helping them develop new attitudes, skills, and ways of relating with each other. When counseling children who have ADHD, therapists should help them learn ways of feeling better about themselves. They should also help the kids identify and work on their strengths besides learning how to cope with problems that they face in their lives. In addition, they should also be taught how to manage their attention and aggression.

Every member of the family is most likely to be affected if one of your kids has ADHD. Consequently, the entire family will need help so that everyone learns how to cope with the condition. Since kids with ADHD often have disruptive behaviors, therapists should focus on finding ways of handling such behaviors. This may entail teaching parents and other family members some techniques for coping with the behaviors and how to improve them.

Psychotherapy doesn't address the underlying causes or symptoms of ADHD. It basically entails the kids and their families talking to the therapist about upsetting feelings and thoughts. This helps them explore self-defeating behavioral patterns besides learning alternative ways of handling their emotions. As family members and parents talk to therapists, they will be able to understand how to deal with the disorder in a better way.

Behavioral therapists help ADHD kids and their families to develop ways of handling immediate issues that may arise. Rather than helping the kids understand their feelings and actions, behavioral therapy helps them change their thinking and, consequently, leads to changes in their behavior. This kind of support to the kids and their family members is akin to practical assistance, which helps them become more organized when undertaking their tasks, besides helping them deal with emotionally-charged events.

On the other hand, social skills training helps children who have ADHD to learn new behaviors. This basically involves therapists discussing with the kids and their families appropriate behaviors that help build and maintain social relationships, such as waiting for a turn, responding to teasing, and asking for help. For instance, the kids might be taught how to read people's facial expressions and voice tones so that they learn how to respond appropriately. Social skills training help family members and the kids themselves develop ways of socializing.

Support groups can be used to help parents connect with other parents whose kids are suffering from ADHD. Support groups members can meet on a regular basis and listen to behavioral experts so that they learn how best to deal with their kids' situation. They also enable parents to share their successes and failures as far as managing ADHD and are a great place to obtain referrals to experts and pertinent information in dealing with ADHD.

Parental skills training is offered either in special classes or behavioral therapists to parents with the objective of giving them techniques for managing their kids' behavior. The most common technique is rewarding good behavior and isolating them when they misbehave. When kids are rewarded for good behavior or completing tasks, they identify desirable behaviors that they should uphold, and undesirable behaviors to avoid. Over time, such techniques help ADHD kids to learn how to control their behavior and thus choose those ones that are desirable.

When handling their ADHD kids, parents also need to learn ways of structuring situations in a manner that allows their kids to succeed. This includes allowing them to interact with several playmates at a time, avoiding overstimulation and situations that will cause them to be hyperactive or impulsive. If your kid has difficulties completing tasks, you can help them learn to do so by dividing large tasks into smaller bits. They should be praised and rewarded as he/she completes the smaller tasks.

Parents should also learn how to use stress management techniques, such as relaxation methods, exercise, and meditation. This will increase their tolerance for frustration, thus enabling them to respond more calmly to their child's behavior.

Home Activities and Simple Exercises for Child with ADHD

Generally, children with ADHD need help to organize their daily activities. In this regard, there are some simple exercises and home activities that come in handy. Treating ADHD starts with scheduling their activities in such a way that they have a similar routine on a daily basis. Spontaneous behavior can be averted if ADHD kids are tuned to adhere to the same routine from the time they wake up until they go to bed. The schedule ought to incorporate activities such as homework time, outdoor recreation, and indoor activities, and should be put somewhere they can easily see to ensure memorization. In case there is any change in the schedule, ensure that the change is communicated to your kids in advance.

Parents and family members should also organize items needed on a daily basis. This will go a long way in preventing spontaneous and unpredictable reactions, which are likely to manifest when ADHD kids fail to find whatever they are looking for. In this regard, you should consider setting aside a place for everything. Besides this, ensure that everything is kept in its place, including school supplies, clothing, and backpacks.

You should also consider using notebook and homework reminders to keep your kids apprised of what he/she should be doing at a particular time. This comes in handy when they are doing school-related chores such as assignments. In line with this, stress to them why it is important to write down all assignments that they are given at school and coming home with the needed books. This way, it will be difficult for them to forget about their assignments. You should take note of the fact that ADHD children need consistent rules that are easy to understand and abide by. If the rules that you lay down for them are followed, ensure that you give appropriate rewards. Always look out for any good behavior that they exhibit and praise it accordingly.

Managing ADHD within the School Environment

The fact that you have a child with ADHD doesn't mean that he/she shouldn't be given an opportunity to attend school. Actually, the social interactions that ADHD kids have at a school, play a significant role as far as behavioral change is concerned. ADHD isn't only managed within the home environment but also at school. Even though you won't be at school with your kid, there are certain measures that you can take to ensure that the disorder is managed within their learning environment.

When it comes to the management of ADHD within the school environment, you should keep in mind the fact that you are your kid's best advocate. To effectively play this role, you need to be as conversant as possible with this behavioral disorder. Learn everything you can about ADHD and the effect that it has on your kid's behavior within the home environment, at school, and in diverse social situations. If your kid has portrayed ADHD symptoms since early on in his/her life, and the disorder has been diagnosed and treated using a combination of behavioral therapy and medical interventions, you should let teachers know about it. This will put them in a position to understand your kid's behavior. Likewise, they will know how best to handle that kid in the new setting, away from the home environment.

In case your child has entered the school system and is having problems that lead you to suspect that he/she has ADHD, it is advisable that you either seek advice from a behavioral expert. Besides this, you can have an evaluation undertaken by the local school district. Generally, schools are mandated to evaluate kids who they suspect to have behavioral disabilities, including ADHD. This is more so the case if the disorder is affecting their academic work and social interactions with teachers and fellow learners. If you think that your school-going ADHD child isn't learning as he/she should make it a point to establish who you need to contact within the school system. Thereafter, you can request that the school undertake an evaluation.

For many years, many schools were reluctant to admit children with ADHD, or even evaluate those already within the system who are suspected of having the disorder. Nevertheless, laws have been made making it mandatory for schools to evaluate kids, in a bid to establish whether their poor academic performance or social skills are caused by behavioral disorders such as ADHD. Once your kid is diagnosed with ADHD, it is obvious that he/she qualifies for specialized educational services. In line with this, the child's school must work with you to assess his/her strengths and weaknesses in view of coming up with an individualized educational program. With such a program in place, it will be easy to gauge the kid's performance even when he/she transitions to a different school.

ADHD and Teenage Transition

As your kid grows older and transitions into a teenager, ADHD stays with him/her. By this time, you should have learned how to manage the symptoms of the disorder as your child proceeds to middle school and, thereafter, junior high. In as much as the child may have been evaluated periodically through the years, it is good practice to undertake another re-evaluation as teenage years set in. Generally, the teenage years are challenging for many children, regardless of whether they have a behavioral disorder or not. Children with ADHD, in particular, find their teenage years even more stressful because, in addition to their condition, they have to battle with typical adolescent problems such as peer pressure, fear of failure in school and socially, and low self-esteem. These, among other challenges, make it hard for ADHD children to cope with adolescence compared to "normal" teens.

Like every teenager, ADHD teens experience the desire to be independent and try new or forbidden things, such as sexual activity, drugs, and alcohol. Needless to say, engaging in such behaviors often leads to undesirable consequences. Owing to the numerous challenges that ADHD teens face, it is advisable that clear rules be laid down and adhered to. Rules meant to guide the behavior of ADHD teens should not only be straightforward but also easy to understand. There also needs to be seamless communication between parents and their teens because, unlike during their younger years, teens can easily express themselves. Therefore, parents should let them understand the reasons behind each rule. These rules should stipulate how teens should behave, both at home and outside the home environment.

Since ADHD adolescents are emotionally fragile, parents ought to respond calmly whenever they break rules. Punishment should be used sparingly and, just like as it is the case with pre-school children, time-outs should be used to control inappropriate behavior. Typically, hot temper and impulsivity accompany ADHD amongst teenagers. Therefore, time alone can help them calm down and return to their senses.

As ADHD teenagers increasingly spend more time away from the home environment, there will be demands such as the use of family cars and later curfews. When such requests are made, listen to them carefully and give concise reasons for your opinions. Learn to negotiate and compromise since this will ultimately prove helpful.

Treatment of ADHD in Adults

Therapy

The idea of ADHD therapy for adults is to help them know how best they can manage their condition. It similarly helps them learn how to change whatever long-standing poor self-image that they might have. They do so by examining their experiences with the disorder in years gone by, and how to avoid the not-so-good ones.

Psychotherapy is often used alongside medical interventions to manage ADHD and its symptoms in adults. You have to keep in mind the fact that even though medication alleviates some of the symptoms of ADHD, individuals ought to make a deliberate effort to sign up for both individual therapy and psycho-education sessions. Psychotherapy for adults' ADHD classes typically entails teaching patients how to embrace their condition without feeling bitter about the impact that it might have had on their lives.

Those who are forgetful can use props and reminders to keep them apprised of their schedules. Likewise, ADHD adults who find it cumbersome to complete tasks can have those tasks broken down into smaller portions. The completion of individual mini-tasks will give them a sense of accomplishment. What's more, it is advisable that adult ADHD individuals learn as much as they can about the disorder since it will put them in a good position to face it.

The success of psychotherapy sessions for ADHD adults starts with them remembering minor routines; keeping the appointment time with the therapist is a good start. This is a step in the right direction and will help them learn how to keep subsequent appointments with the therapists and any other people that they are to meet in future.

In most cases, therapists encourage ADHD adults who are seeking treatment to adjust to whatever changes that the therapy sessions might have brought to their lives. Such changes may include the apparent loss of impulsivity, a diminished love for risk-taking, and the new sense of thinking before making any decisions. Such changes are likely to be worrisome to some patients and, therefore, the therapist needs to explain this to them once they start experiencing the changes. As adult ADHD patients begin experiencing minor success in their ability to organize what would hitherto be complex situations, it becomes easy for them to appreciate and embrace ADHD characteristics that are positive. These include boundless warmth, energy, and enthusiasm.

Risks of Untreated Adult ADHD

Like has been mentioned earlier, ADHD in adults often remains undetected in most cases. Untreated ADHD among both kids and adults tends to lead to a myriad of problems throughout one's life. Due to the impulsiveness and short attention spans that characterize individuals with ADHD, leaving the condition unattended makes it hard for them to succeed in school, climb the career ladder, and build strong relationships. Simply put, the disorder affects all aspects of an individual's life if it is left untreated.

Adults who have ADHD that is undetected and untreated often find it difficult to manage their emotions and ensuing reactions. As a result, they end up experiencing social problems, since they may not know how best to take turns, interact with others, or even react appropriately in certain situations. Without treatment and therapy, their social circle may be limited to close family members' due to a lack of the ability to make and keep friends. Many people unknowingly regard ADHD adults as being hard to deal with. In the end, they shun them, something that often leads such individuals to suffer from depression and a lack of self-esteem.

Adults who have untreated ADHD are also more likely to get into car accidents, be in trouble with the law, or have gambling problems due to impulsivity. Research indicates that up to 40% of prison inmates have a form of ADHD. In most of these cases, the disorder is either undiagnosed or untreated. This clearly suggests that had these individuals been diagnosed and treated for ADHD early enough, actions that led to their incarceration may not have occurred in the first place.

How Long Should ADHD Medication be Administered?

The amount of time that ADHD medication is administered generally depends on the severity of the disorder and the potency of the drug being used. In children, teens, and college students, it is recommended that ADHD medication is administered throughout their school year so that they can concentrate better in class.

Beyond college, the length of treatment will depend on an individual's situation and the level of general pressure from external factors such as work, home, or in social situations, and how they are handling them. Whether one stays on medication at all times is a personal decision. You have to keep in mind that assists ADHD patients maintain whatever positive improvements they may have made in their lives. This way, it will be possible for them to keep making positive and meaningful changes going forward.

Most patients who seek treatment for ADHD often seek interventions for disorders that go beyond ADHD. This is why it is advisable to combine medication and therapy, or any other non-pharmacological interventions that a medical practitioner may deem fit. In most cases, the baggage that accompanies ADHD is usually part of the problem and, therefore, doctors must also focus on the. A significant number of emotional issues that most ADHD patients experience have something to do with them feeling bad about themselves and that they feel incapable of being competent. The situation is compounded by the fact that before ADHD gets diagnosed, many patients receive negative feedback from their friends, colleagues, and family members who typically consider them to be lazy and not good enough.

Should Patients Consider Psychotherapy?

Talking therapy and cognitive-behavioral therapy should be part and parcel of ADHD treatment. This intervention is particularly recommended to adults who have ADHD since it will help them hone their organizational skills. If someone has a history of other mental issues, they should consider talking therapy. If ADHD is the primary behavioral disorder, the doctor will probably focus on enhancing executive functions, which include organizational skills, time management, and planning.

Therapy for ADHD also involves helping patients to gain more mastery over their emotions and reactions. Behavioral therapy with specific goals can address the symptoms and behaviors that are deemed to be detrimental and problematic. For instance, patients who have difficulties keeping to appointments certainly have problems with planning their time. To remedy this, the therapist will try finding ways through which that patient can learn how to maintain a calendar. The success of therapy is hinged on the ability of the practitioner to help patients make changes in their lives, unlearn bad habits, plan better, react to situations in a more appropriate manner, and listen better.

ADHD Coaching

In recent years, there has been the emergence of ADHD coaching. This intervention not only offers specific problem-solving but also works effectively for severe cases. ADHD is akin to situations where there is a learner and a tutor, and involves working on specific issues that a patient might be experiencing. Pairing ADHD patients with coaches for sessions of up to 8 weeks improves their organizational ability, besides reducing anger levels that most of them might have maintained for up to a year.

Generally, ADHD coaching targets specific areas of weaknesses, including low motivation, poor organizational skills, impulsivity, poor anger control, and attention problems. When these specific problems are addressed, it is easy to put patients back on track. Most coaches who offer ADHD coaching are not therapists or medical experts. Personal coaching helps patients to understand both the nature of ADHD and the impact that the condition had in their lives. Similarly, it helps patients learn ways of facing obstacles and focus on their goals. Coaches work with patients to create strategies, structures, and build skills that help them address ADHD-related issues such as organization, self-esteem, and time management. Therefore, you should only choose one who has a history of working with ADHD patients.

Can ADHD Be Treated Without Drugs?

The short answer to this is, "yes." Once a positive ADHD diagnosis has been made, the long trek through the pharmaceutical world begins. Medication is the preferred intervention for ADHD since it is effective for up to 80% of patients. When ADHD is diagnosed, many people start worrying about the medication side effects. On paper, these look scary and, therefore, patients and their family members often prefer exhausting other ADHD treatment before medication is considered.

In children, it is recommended that medication only starts after they start going to school. Before that, behavioral therapy should be used instead of drugs. Quite often, patients inquire whether they can try out other treatments before they consider medicine. When mitigating the symptoms of ADHD in kids, it is always advisable for parents to find out about other treatments that work for their kids before they turn to medication. Behavioral therapy alone can be effective, especially in pre-school kids who are only showing unfocused and inattentive symptoms. In older kids and adults, a combination of medicine and behavioral treatment works best.

Alternative Interventions to Medicines and Therapy

Apart from medicine and therapy, there are other interventions that can help to manage symptoms of ADHD, and for the individual to live a "normal" life. For instance, getting enough sleep can be beneficial to kids with ADHD since it particularly helps with impulsivity and restlessness.

Sleep

Most kids who have ADHD also suffer from sleep disorders. In such cases, the presence of each disorder makes the other even worse. The most common sleep disorder for children with ADHD is the inability to settle down, preventing them from falling asleep. They end up experiencing exhaustion the following day, something that makes them even more restless. While some medical practitioners recommend the use of sleeping aids, such as melatonin, parents should start with practicing good sleep habits. This includes having consistent bedtime routines even on weekends, keeping kids' bedrooms dark, and creating a calming winding-down ritual every night.

Exercise

Plenty of exercise can also help both ADHD adults and children to manage their symptoms more effectively. In this regard, there's a need for patients to have plenty of opportunities for exercising at appropriate times. Research indicates that up to 30 minutes of exercise helps kids who have ADHD to be more focused and organized in their activities. Water has a natural calming effect, and so swimming can be a very popular form of exercise for people with ADHD thus having a knock-on calming effect to other areas of their lives.

Exercise isn't only good for keeping the body fit. It also helps maintain brain health. Whenever you exercise, the brain releases neurotransmitters such as dopamine, which enhances clear thinking and attention. Individuals who have ADHD often tend to have low levels of dopamine in their brains. Exercising helps ease anxiety and stress, both in ADHD kids and adults. It also improves impulse control, thus reducing compulsive behavior.

Those with ADHD who regularly exercise also have improved working memory and enhanced executive function. This enables them to plan and organize their activities more effectively, besides remembering specific details. Exercising also increases the level of the brain-derived neurotropic factor, a protein that enhances memory and learning, and is usually in short supply among individuals who are suffering from ADHD.

Meditation and Mindfulness

Recent studies have unraveled that mindfulness and meditation can help individuals with ADHD cope better with the disorder. Mindfulness and meditation typically involve learning how to become more aware, sharpen focus, and practice self-control through breathing. When those with ADHD complete a mindfulness training program, they are likely to exhibit fewer symptoms of the disorder. Meditation can also control impulsivity because patients learn to control their thoughts before doing anything.

Meditation can go a long way in counteracting the stress of an adrenaline rush. When the word "meditation" is mentioned, many people who have ADHD may think that it can never apply to them. Meditation is among the most effective self-help techniques that can help people with ADHD stay calm. Meditation generally involves observing your moment-to-moment feelings and thoughts, with the objective of calming your mind and improving your focus. Unlike other treatments used to manage the symptoms of ADHD, meditation doesn't require any prescription, nor those seemingly endless trips to a therapist's office; you can meditate from the comfort of your bedroom.

Just the same way that we exercise to strengthen a specific part of our bodies, mindful meditation seeks to strengthen your ability to manage your reactions. It, similarly, helps you control your attention. If done correctly, it will help you learn ways of observing yourself and focus on a desired result. Mindful meditation itself is quite easy and doesn't require the presence of a guru.

Contrary to information that has been peddled in the public domain, meditation is easy, and you can't fail at it. You only need to get comfortable, find your comfort zone, and tone down from your full, high-speed adrenaline mode. Meditation trains you to control your wandering mind and bring it back to the moment before you become distracted. What's more, it makes you aware of your emotions, thus making you less vulnerable to impulsive behavior. It also raises the level of dopamine in your body, which is usually in short supply in individuals who have ADHD. Simply put, mindful meditation is an impulse control strategy.

Apart from mindful meditation, yoga can also be used to manage the often destructive symptoms of hyperactive-impulsive ADHD. It also increased dopamine levels in the brain, as well as strengthening the prefrontal cortex. A study among ADHD kids and adults established that those who practice yoga 20 minutes twice weekly for eight weeks made a significant improvement in their focus and attention, something that put them a better position to handle their condition. The use of mindful meditation and yoga to manage the symptoms of ADHD may look like an unexpected match but nonetheless, it significantly improves brain executive functions such as attention, concentration, and memory.

Recommended Food & Supplements to help with ADHD

Apart from medicine, therapy, and exercise, there are a number of foods and supplements that can help ADHD patients fight off detrimental symptoms. Some of the so-called alternative treatments for ADHD are inexpensive, easy to administer, and relatively safe, without side effects. However, the indicating that work faces strong arguments that this isn't the case. It is just the same with existing claims that sugar causes ADHD. Much controversy surrounding the link between sugar and ADHD still exists. The main question is whether or not sugar leads to hyperactivity. In as much as there is no proof to show that sugar leads to hyperactivity, many people still wonder why individuals seem to become hyperactive when they consume sugar in significant quantities.

Supplements Used to Manage ADHD Symptoms

1. Zinc

Some studies have suggested that kids who have ADHD have low zinc levels in their bodies. Zinc, which helps to enhance brain health, is one of the most essential minerals. Zinc deficiency not only affects other nutrients but also impacts on the brain function. Incorporating zinc-based supplements alleviates the symptoms of impulsivity, hyperactivity, and social problems, which characterize those with ADHD. Therefore, it can be said that taking zinc supplements can go a long way in improving some of the symptoms that ADHD individuals exhibit. Foods that are rich in zinc include seafood, poultry, red meat, beans, nuts, dairy products, fortified cereals, and whole grains.

2. Omega-3 Fatty Acids

There is proof that eating a diet rich in omega-3 fatty acids can improve ADHD symptoms. This supplement can be found in fish oil, and helps enhance the mental coordination of those with ADHD especially kids. They also ought to improve the ability to organize and plan. Vayarin, an FDA-approved supplement, is the most common and widely-used omega-3 fatty acid used by those with ADHD.

3. Iron

Some studies have attempted to link ADHD with low iron levels. One such study has proved that iron deficiency increases the risk of mental disorders among kids and young adults. Iron is essential in the production of dopamine and norepinephrine, which are neurotransmitters that regulate emotions, stress, and the brain's reward system. According to medical practitioners, iron supplements can help relieve the symptoms of ADHD, especially in people who have an iron deficiency. It's important that there's an awareness surrounding the toxicity of over consuming iron. Therefore, a doctor should be consulted prior to taking iron supplements.

4. Magnesium

This is an important mineral that contributes significantly to brain health. Magnesium deficiency causes mental confusion, shortened attention span, and irritability however; you might not notice the benefits of supplementation if you're not magnesium deficient. Just like the case with iron, it is important to consult a doctor before you embark on the use of magnesium. When used in high doses, this supplement can lead to diarrhea, cramps, and nausea.

Herbs for ADHD

In recent years, there has been a growing popularity for the use of herbal remedies to manage ADHD symptoms. Just because herbal remedies are natural, it doesn't automatically mean that they are effective when compared to traditional treatments.

The following are some of the herbal remedies used to treat ADHD.

1. Korean Ginseng

An observational study meant to establish the effectiveness of Korean ginseng on children with ADHD established that the herb significantly reduces hyperactive behavior.

2. Valerian Root

It has been found that this herb can significantly increase concentration in ADHD individuals by up to 50% while decreasing hyperactivity. It also decreases impulsiveness while improving social behavior and sleep. These findings make it an effective treatment alongside other interventions.

ADHD Diets

There is no scientific proof that ADHD is caused by nutritional or diet problems. Nevertheless, research indicates that some foods may play a role in worsening or improving the symptoms of ADHD. Your eating habits go a long way in helping the brain function better. This, in turn, lessens typical ADHD symptoms such as a lack of focus and restlessness.

Generally, the main assumption that exists as far as the ADHD diet is concerned is that some of the foods that we eat either make ADHD symptoms better or worse. Elimination diets have also become popular. This mainly entails avoiding foods or ingredients that might trigger certain ADHD-related behaviors, thus worsening symptoms. For example, some flavorings, colorings, and preservatives increase hyperactivity among kids. The American Academy of Pediatrics states that eliminating some food colorings and preservatives can go a long way in mitigating some symptoms of hyperactive-impulsive ADHD.

The main consensus that exists when it comes to ADHD diets is that any food that is good for the brain improves the symptoms of ADHD. Therefore, you should consider eating high-protein diets comprising items such as beans, meat, cheese, and nuts, since they improve concentration, aside from helping certain medicine to work better.

It is also advisable to consume fewer simple carbohydrates such as candy, corn, and sugar since they are thought to increase hyperactivity. On the flipside, it is advisable to increase the intake of complex carbohydrates such as oranges, pears, tangerines, apples, grapefruit, and kiwi since they improve sleep, as well as reducing anxiety.

Chapter 5: ADHD and Other Mental Disorders

ADHD With Learning Disabilities in a Child

Many parents have been mistakenly led to believe that ADHD is a type of learning disability. This could be perhaps attributed to the fact that generally, the two disorders occur concurrently. Up to 30% of kids who have ADHD have a form of a learning disorder. According to child psychiatrists, having either of the conditions makes the other likely to occur, too. Thus, it goes without saying that ADHD can lead to learning difficulties in children. This is attested the fact that typically, ADHD children find it hard to focus in class and other activities for long enough. They similarly have trouble following instructions and directions. This doesn't however, mean that ADHD is a learning disability.

The distinctions between ADHD and learning difficulties have been shifting. In as much as the two disorders largely overlap, each has its own diagnostic criteria. Generally, there are several learning disabilities, and a child may have more than one of these. When either a parent or teacher suspects that a child has a learning disability, a psycho-educational test must be immediately conducted to confirm it. This test basically evaluates kids' intelligence or ability versus their achievement on standardized tests. Children who have learning disabilities often have average or above average IQ, however, often encounter difficulties when it comes to the processing and retrieval of information. This explains why they don't perform well in school tests.

Just like learning difficulties, ADHD also affects kids' ability to learn. Children who have ADHD have a number of brain function impairments, which makes them hyperactive, inattentive, or impulsive. As a result, these kids may seem to have learning difficulties simply because they are often hampered from acquiring working skills and information due to either their hyperactive behavior or inattentiveness.

What Are Some of the Most Common Learning Disabilities?

The most prevalent learning disabilities, which often get confused with ADHD, are:

- **Dyslexia.** This language disability mainly hinders kids' ability to understand and process written words. In some cases, dyslexia is referred to as a reading disability/disorder.

- **Dyscalculia.** Just like the name suggests, dyscalculia is a learning disability that makes it hard for kids to learn how to work out mathematical problems or grasp mathematical concepts.

- **Dysgraphia.** This learning disability is characterized by the inability to write. Children who have this disorder struggle to write or even form letters within a specified space.

- **Visual processing and auditory disorders.** A child who has these sensory disorders often struggles to understand language despite the fact that their senses of vision and hearing are normal.

- **Nonverbal Disabilities. These are typical neurological disorders, which often lead to difficulties in intuition, organization, spatial relations, and evaluation.**

What is the Connection Between Learning Difficulties and ADHD?

Dyslexia is the most common learning disorder in children. Research indicates that 15 to 20% of kids who have ADHD also suffer from a reading disability which is twice the average. In addition, impairments in the social, emotional, and academic areas of functioning are worse when a kid is affected by both ADHD and a learning difficulty. In the event that a kid is affected by a specific learning difficulty, there is a need to distinguish it from the attention and behavioral aspects of ADHD.

Tips to Overcome Learning Difficulties and ADHD

Since the possibility of a child with ADHD to also have a learning disability is high, there is a need for both disorders to be treated. The two disorders should be concurrently treated to attain the most desired outcome. For instance, if a child is being treated for ADHD, chances are high that their learning disability will persist. Likewise, if they are receiving assistance to treat their learning difficulty, the desired outcome possibly won't be attained if their problems of a lack of focus and impulsivity aren't addressed.

Generally, ADHD kids qualify to receive specialized education as stipulated by the Individuals with Disabilities Education Act. Children who have ADHD, or any learning disability, are legally entitled to, and can benefit from an individualized education program that is designed to address their learning needs. Therefore, parents, guidance counselors, and teachers ought to work in tandem to form an IEP (individualized education program) before kids start school. The program needs to be regularly updated to accommodate the kids' emerging educational needs. In as much as neither learning disabilities nor ADHD can fully be cured, a kid can still live with the disorders and have a happy and successful life.

ADHD with Autism Spectrum Disorder in a Child and an Adult

Autism Spectrum Disorder (ASD) is a mental condition which makes the interaction and communication with others difficult. Kids and adults who have autism often face significant challenges. Typical symptoms that they exhibit can be: an inability to understand others' feelings, poor communication skills, delays in motor skills, poor understanding of abstract language uses such as conversation and humor, obsessive interest in certain information or items, and strong reaction to senses and stimuli.

On the other hand, ADHD is characterized by difficulties in paying attention, sitting still, and the tendency to act impulsively. The fourth edition of DSM-IV stipulated that both ADHD and ASD can't be co-diagnosed. However, DSM-5 recognized that the two disorders are interrelated and that both adults and kids can be affected concurrently by the two. Recently, DSM-5 was changed to eliminate the exclusion of the dual diagnosis of both ASD and ADHD.

Studies indicate that up to 29% of ASD kids aged between 4 and 8 years also exhibit some of the most common symptoms of ADHD. Moreover, adults and kids who have comorbid ADHD and ASD have significantly lower cognitive functioning, severe social impairment, and significant delays in adaptive functioning compared to children and adults who have ASD only. This shows that the presence of ADHD in kids and adults who have ASD greatly complicate their learning and understanding. Parents and family members of children and adults who have both conditions also report that those affected tend to have repetitive and stereotypical behaviors compared to those who either have ADHD or ASD alone.

Generally, behaviors that are associated with ASD tend to look like ADHD. This is why most of the symptoms of ASD and ADHD overlap. Kids and adults who suffer from ASD also have symptoms that typify ADHD. These include social awkwardness, an inability to stay calm, and impulsivity. Nevertheless, ADHD in its purest form isn't part of ASD.

What is the Difference Between ADHD and Autism?

Generally, ADHD is characterized by hyperactivity, inattention, and impulsivity. Therefore, the disorder inherently causes problems with executive function and self-regulation. On the other hand, Autism Spectrum Disorders are a continuum of disorders that include Asperger's syndrome, pervasive developmental disorder, and autism. These disorders are typified by problems when it comes to communication, social interactions, and repetitive mannerisms.

Children and adults who have autism don't intuitively understand some of the aspects of the social world that exists around them. As a result, their social development, which is mirrored in their communication and interaction abilities, is greatly delayed. Besides this, these individuals exhibit specific symptoms including poor gesture language and limited imaginative play.

Even though the inherent components of both ASD and ADHD differ, there are a number of overlaps as far as the symptoms of the two disorders are concerned. The main trick as far as distinguishing the two conditions apart, is determining the exact developmental building block or executive function that is missing and thus causing the symptom. Generally, those battling with ADHD may struggle socially. With ADHD alone, proof of early social development, such as turn-taking play, responding to names, imaginative play, and gesture language usually remains intact. Traits such as displaying facial expressions, empathy, and humor also remain unaffected.

When these traits are lacking, it is an indicator that an individual could be autistic. Kids and adults who have ADHD may not have the patience to wait in line but, they understand the concept. They also may not have the ability to respond when called as a result of inattention, but even so, they still remain socially engaged besides recognizing their names.

Diagnosing ASD and ADHD

If both ASD and ADHD are suspected in adults or children, it is advisable that a diagnosis is undertaken by a specialist who is familiar with the two disorders. A thorough examination should be done with the aim of defining the strengths and weaknesses of the affected individuals. Various tests should be carried out to document ADHD and ASD symptoms so that a clear distinction between the two can be made. Tests alone aren't sufficient since the evaluation of both autism and ADHD is a clinical skill, which is based heavily on getting to understand those who are affected by seeking a comprehensive picture of their lives and interactions in the real world. This will give the specialist an insight into the child's/adult's conversational and social skill, as well as their daily living or play skills.

Diagnosing ADHD and ASD can be a fluid and ongoing process rather than a one-off procedure. This is because those affected may initially exhibit ASD-like symptoms only for them to exhibit ADHD symptoms later on. You have to keep in mind the fact that, for people who have co-existing ASD and ADHD, treating either of the conditions first is a means to an end, which is treating the other. Few patients who have both ASD and ADHD succeed in life without medication.

Tips to Overcome ASD and ADHD Comorbidity

Just like it is the case with ADHD and learning difficulties,

ADHD and ASD ought to be treated concurrently. Generally, the interventions used for both ASD and ADHD can help professionals make the most accurate diagnosis. For instance, ADHD medication can help quell the symptoms of the disorder and, in the process, make ASD symptoms clearer. For ADHD, there is substantial proof in favor of the use of medication and therapy to manage symptoms. For autism alone, there are medications that can help minimize specific symptoms, such as obsessive behavior. In either case, the underlying condition won't be treated; only their symptoms.

Non-medical interventions can also be used to help individuals who are suspected of having both ASD and ADHD before they receive a definite diagnosis. If those affected are experiencing ongoing social challenges, for instance, most of the interventions that will be used will be similar. This may include behavioral therapy to help them develop their social skills. To overcome the conditions, counseling and assistance ought to be offered to help those who are affected improve their social and organizational skills. Therapy will also help them grasp whatever gaps that exist between them and society. Other non-medical interventions, such as speech therapy, occupational therapy, parental training, and educational interventions, should also be explored.

ADHD With Anxiety

Anxiety often accompanies ADHD. Chances are high that if someone has been diagnosed with ADHD, they will also suffer from anxiety. Sometimes, anxiety is masked by the more prominent symptoms of ADHD. Nearly half of adults who have ADHD and 30% of kids with ADHD also suffer from an anxiety disorder. Typically, it is difficult to recognize even the most common symptoms of anxiety if you have ADHD. The behavioral disorder is a lifelong condition, which tends to mask other comorbid conditions that accompany it.

ADHD may make you feel uneasy, distressed, and excessively frightened in regular or benign circumstances. Those who have an anxiety disorder may exhibit symptoms that are so severe to the extent that their daily activities including work and study get compromised. In addition, they find it difficult to enjoy their social interactions and relationships. The inherent symptoms of an anxiety disorder differ from those of ADHD. Primarily, ADHD symptoms involve issues pertaining to concentration and focus. On the other hand, anxiety symptoms involve issues that touch on nervousness and fear.

Each of these conditions has its own unique symptoms, with some crossing over to the other. This may make it hard for someone to tell the difference between the two disorders. Just like individuals who are battling with ADHD, those who suffer from an anxiety disorder tend to feel restless all the time, something that renders them unable to relax. Symptoms that are common in individuals suffering from an anxiety disorder alone include a chronic feeling of worry, fear without an obvious or plausible cause, irritability, insomnia, headaches or belly aches, and the fear of trying new things. Some of these symptoms are exhibited by individuals suffering from the various types of ADHD. For instance, children who have hyperactive-impulsive ADHD often have trouble sleeping. Likewise, inattentive type ADHD is sometimes exhibited by the fear of trying new things, especially those that seem to demand mental effort.

Differentiating Between Anxiety and ADHD

Even though a professional assessment is necessary to diagnose whether an individual is battling with both anxiety and ADHD, family members can easily tell the dissimilarities between the two conditions. The secret lies in watching how symptoms of the disorders play out over time. In case you are suffering from anxiety disorder, you may find it difficult to concentrate in circumstances that make you feel anxious. Conversely, those who have ADHD often find it difficult to concentrate most of the time regardless of the situation that they are in.

If you are battling with both ADHD and anxiety disorder, it's likely that the symptoms of both behavioral disorders will seem more extreme. For instance, anxiety may make it even harder for individuals who have ADHD to follow instructions or follow through tasks to the end.

In as much as comorbidity exists between these disorders, it isn't clear why there is a link between anxiety and ADHD. Researchers are yet to pinpoint what exactly causes the two disorders. To some extent, genetics may be responsible for these conditions, and may also lead to comorbidity. Often after ADHD has been diagnosed, anxiety typically sets in, particularly among adults because the condition gives them a lot to worry about. ADHD often causes individuals to utter inappropriate or offensive words without meaning to. In the process, they start worrying about their next move because they fear it might lead to offending others, and even with the law. Worrying too much about what might happen can lead to an anxiety disorder.

What is the Connection Between Anxiety and ADHD?

Most people who are diagnosed with ADHD tend to struggle with time-management skills, organizational skills, and working memory. This makes it hard for them to follow even the simplest of routines or complete long-term tasks. The ridicule that they receive for failing to undertake simple tasks often leads to chronic stress and worry. Children and adults who are suffering from ADHD also end up having problems with emotional regulation. In most cases, they become flooded with both positive and negative emotions, which are often difficult to manage. Ultimately, they end up struggling to make sense of their thoughts, and they also tend to get trapped in a web of anxious and negative thinking.

Since anxiety symptoms tend to mimic ADHD symptoms in both kids and adults, it is easy for a misdiagnosis to occur. This highlights the importance of ensuring that an accurate diagnosis is made via a thorough examination by a neuropsychologist. Anxiety may look like ADHD among kids. Therefore, it is advisable to have a kid assessed by a professional so that the best course of treatment is determined. In as much as the symptoms of ADHD and anxiety may overlap, you should take note of the fact that anxious children tend to exhibit more perfectionist behaviors without worrying about interacting with others. On the other hand, kids who have ADHD tend to struggle with organization and impulse control.

Diagnosis shouldn't be a one-off process. A complete neuropsychological assessment, including a classroom evaluation for kids, will help the specialist determine whether the child's behavior is entrenched in anxiety, ADHD, or a combination of the two disorders.

Tips to Overcome ADHD and Anxiety Disorder Comorbidity

If an individual is displaying symptoms of both anxiety and ADHD, it is advisable to treat both disorders. Treatment needs to be done by a mental health professional. Here are some tips for overcoming ADHD and anxiety disorder:

Understand Your Triggers

Usually, the symptoms of ADHD and anxiety are triggered by specific circumstances. These may include simple situations such as being asked to speak in public. It is advisable to identify situations that trigger anxiety and the symptoms of ADHD. Once these triggers have been identified, one should work with a mental health professional to establish ways of dealing with the symptoms and anxiety, when faced with these situations. For instance, preparing notes to practice a presentation can go a long way in helping someone feel less anxious when speaking in front of an audience.

To manage anxiety in kids, it is also recommended to identify the exact stressors that make them feel anxious. This will help them learn how to foretell anxiety-inducing situations and as a result, he/she will be able to handle the symptoms as they occur.

Get Ample Rest

Tiredness and insufficient sleep increase the risk of feeling anxious. To counter sleep-induced anxiety, it is advisable that an individual sleeps for 7 to 8 hours per night. If someone has trouble falling asleep due to hyperactivity, meditating before bedtime to calm the mind will help. In addition, one should try going to bed and waking up at the same time each day.

In cases where medication is being taken for ADHD or anxiety, chances are high that it could be affecting sleep. In this case, an additional sleep aid, albeit temporarily, may be required. Avoid taking additional anxiety or sleep medication without consulting a doctor since it can make ADHD or anxiety symptoms even worse. Besides having sufficient sleep and rest, it is also good to exercise regularly.

Create a Schedule

If someone is suffering from ADHD, the completion of tasks may be a tall order. In most people, this makes their anxiety even worse. To avoid such a situation, it is advisable that you to create a schedule that will guide important and daily activities. Sticking to this schedule will help in their completion, without having to forget any. If ADHD exists, a person should avoid burdening or stressing themselves out about completing their tasks within schedule. Instead, they should expect for each task to take longer than the time allocated towards it. Setting unrealistic goals will only but worsen the anxiety.

Keep a Journal

There is no better way of suppressing anxiety than writing down what you feel about it. Writing a journal is one of the best ways of doing this since it clears your mind, besides enabling you to focus on what you are doing at that particular point. In addition, a journal makes you more committed towards your treatment, particularly if you develop the habit of going through it. To keep a journal, you must feel comfortable enough to write down whatever is on your mind at any particular time. This will help you pinpoint any issues that you would ultimately want to discuss with your therapist or doctor during your next visit.

Practice Thought Stopping

Thought stopping can be used to manage anxiety, especially within children. Generally, ADHD kids who also suffer from anxiety struggle with thought flooding. The anxious thoughts that flood their mind all at once often overwhelm them. Recovering from this is difficult because of the intricate pattern of anxious thinking. To prevent this situation, the children should be taught to practice thought stopping. During their calmest moments, have the kids practice telling themselves, "No brain, stop saying that to me. I can handle this." When kids learn to "talk back" to whatever is worrying them, it becomes easy for them to replace their anxious thoughts with more positive ones. It similarly becomes easy for them to interrupt the worry cycle whenever it creeps up, and to reset themselves accordingly. This also applies to adults who are battling ADHD and anxiety.

Deep Breathing

Breathing deeply is a tested and proven strategy for fighting anxiety, both in children and adults. Deep breathing not only slows down your heart-beat but also helps to relieve muscle tension. When individuals suffering from ADHD learn to deep breathe whenever worrying thoughts come up, they gain the ability to stay relaxed, thus dispelling such thoughts. With time, they develop the ability to handle their anxious thoughts accordingly and replace negative and anxious thinking with peaceful thinking.

Psychotherapy

Psychotherapy is one strategy that works for nearly all mental and behavioral disorders. If ADHD and comorbid anxiety impact daily life, career progression, and social interactions, psychotherapy from a mental health professional can really help. Through psychotherapy, ADHD kids and adults who are also suffering from anxiety will be able to manage their emotions. Besides this, they will develop the ability to identify stressors and anxiety triggers.

ADHD With Depression

ADHD and depression often go hand in hand since they tend to co-exist at the same time. Whereas ADHD affects an individual's ability to focus, depression is more than an infrequent case of the blues. This condition is characterized by a deep feeling of despair and sadness, which may last up to two weeks at a time. Depression may make it hard for you to attend to your daily duties or even fall asleep. Up to 30% of kids who have ADHD also suffer from a serious mood disorder. In addition, more than half of individuals who have ADHD get treated for depression at some point.

What is the Link Between ADHD and Depression?

Some of the most prominent symptoms of depression and ADHD are similar. This may make it hard to diagnose the conditions and treat them accordingly. For instance, those suffering from ADHD or depression may also have trouble with focus. If you take medication to aid with the ADHD symptom, your sleep or appetite is likely to be affected. Needless to say, these can also be symptoms of depression. In kids, irritability and hyperactivity are symptoms of ADHD as well as depression.

ADHD can also cause depression, especially in instances when those who are affected have trouble managing their symptoms. For instance, kids may have trouble when it comes to getting along with their peers at school or when playing. Likewise, adults may also have deep-seated issues at work. This can lead to a deep feeling of hopelessness, which is a common symptom of depression. In as much as medical practitioners cannot point out the exact cause of both depression and ADHD, the two conditions seem to be related to an individual's family history. Individuals who have ADHD or depression often have a family member who also has it.

Studies show that up to 70% of individuals suffering from ADHD have sought treatment for depression at some point. Teens who have ADHD are 10 times more likely to also suffer from depression, compared to those who do not have ADHD. Whereas boys are more likely to battle ADHD in their lives, girls have a higher risk of suffering from depression alongside ADHD. Children who get diagnosed with ADHD when they are young are similarly at a higher risk of developing depression.

Generally, individuals who have the inattentive type of ADHD are at a higher risk of depression compared to those battling with either the combination type of ADHD or the hyperactive-impulsive ADHD type.

Typically, individuals who have ADHD tend to experience mood swings that are triggered by certain events or circumstances. This is not the case among those suffering from depression, because their low mood may even last for months. Just like other mental disorders that are comorbid with ADHD, the main challenge when diagnosing depression and/or ADHD is the overlapping symptoms. These include feeling restless and experiencing difficulties in concentrating.

To compound the situation, most side effects of ADHD medications, such as insomnia and fatigue, tend to imitate depressive episodes. This highlights the significance of speaking to a psychiatrist, so that the exact cause of whatever symptoms are experienced, get pinpointed.

What Are the Distinguishing Symptoms Between ADHD and Depression?

Certain symptoms can be used to determine whether a patient is suffering from depression, ADHD, or both. Assessing these symptoms can go a long way in eliminating the confusion that exists as far as diagnosing ADHD and depression is concerned. Needless to say, differentiating these two disorders can be hard, owing to the fact that both lead to forgetfulness, mood problems, lack of motivation, and an inability to focus.

There are a number of subtle distinctions between symptoms caused by depression and ADHD-induced symptoms.

- **Emotions.** ADHD can lead to low moods. These episodes are usually caused by specific setbacks.

Moreover, the dark moods that ADHD patients may experience are usually transient in nature. On the other hand, the low mood issues that are linked to depression are pervasive and generally chronic in nature. They may last for weeks or months at a time. Unlike the low moods that are caused by ADHD which begin in childhood, depression doesn't usually develop until one reaches his/her teenage years.

- **Motivation.** When it comes to ADHD, it often seems impossible to complete any task. This comes about simply because those who are affected tend to dither without deciding which task they should tackle first. With depression, there is no uncertainty in the first place, patients are too lethargic to the extent that they cannot initiate any activity.

- **Sleep Problems.** With ADHD, individuals often experience problems once they get to bed. Due to their hyperactive nature, the minds of such individuals tend to simply refuse to "turn off." This contrasts sharply from people who are suffering from depression. They may instantly fall asleep as soon as they get to bed but they tend to sleep intermittently. Whenever they wake up repeatedly at night, their minds tend to be filled with anxious or negative thoughts.

Tips to Overcome Depression With ADHD

The most effective way of overcoming depression with ADHD is the use of medication, in order to quell the symptoms of each disorder. Even though these conditions tend to occur at the same time, one of them is likely to cause a greater impairment. You have to keep in mind the fact that even though problems caused by ADHD are real and serious, depression is a life-threatening disorder. Antidepressants that boost the level and performance of neurotransmitters can be used to remedy severe cases of ADHD with depression. In mild to moderate cases of depression with ADHD, an antidepressant can also be prescribed.

Most antidepressants are effective when used alongside ADHD stimulant and non-stimulant medication. Nearly half of individuals who take antidepressants to manage the symptoms of ADHD often end up achieving complete relief from symptoms of depression.

Apart from treatment, psychotherapy can effectively be used to treat depression with ADHD. The most efficient form of psychotherapy for use in this regard is cognitive behavioral therapy (CBT). This form of therapy mainly entails identifying the types of negative and anxious thoughts that individuals experience, and their frequency. Thereafter, work is done with the therapist to replace these self-destructive beliefs and thoughts with realistic thoughts. A negative thought such as "this is hard," will have to be replaced by a constructive one like, "Yes, this is hard, but I can manage." In as much as the difficulty of the task, you acknowledged, such a thought shows that the individual isn't wallowing in its difficulty. Instead, the direction is shifted to positive action for tackling that difficulty.

The objective of psychotherapy should be to minimize the intensity and frequency of not only the negative thoughts but also the symptoms of ADHD with depression.

You can also use meditation to treat depression that accompanies ADHD. For optimum results, sit in a quiet room with closed eyes. When doing this, focus solely on breathing while repeating a familiar word. It could be a spouse's name or a letter in the alphabet. Do this for 10-20 seconds every time a feeling of depressions sets in can go a long way in helping control ADHD and coexisting depression.

ADHD With Bipolar Disorder

It goes without saying that dealing with ADHD is a major challenge. Throw in bipolar disorder and it becomes even harder. It is difficult to distinguish between ADHD and bipolar disorder among kids and adults since both conditions have similar symptoms.

In its purest form, bipolar disorder is typified by mood swings between periods of extreme highs and lows. Bipolar in children is often a somewhat chronic mood deregulation characterized by a mix of elation, irritability, and depression.

There are certain symptoms that are present in kids suffering from both bipolar disorder and ADHD. These include a decreased need for sleep and high energy levels. In adults, bipolar disorder and ADHD tend to occur together. Between 15 and 17% of individuals who have bipolar disorder also suffer from ADHD. A clear distinction between the two conditions can be made owing to the fact that ADHD is characterized by the triad of impulsivity, restlessness, and distractibility. These symptoms must be present consistently and must also cause one form of impairment or another throughout an individual's life.

Bipolar disorder and ADHD can be differentiated by these pertinent factors:

- **Age of onset.** Generally, ADHD symptoms manifest themselves throughout an individual's lifetime. These symptoms ought to be present, though not necessarily impairing, by the age of 7. On its part, bipolar disorder can be present in preteens but even so, symptoms of the disorder tend to be so rare that researchers say it doesn't occur.

- **Consistency of symptoms and impairment.** ADHD remains present even when its symptoms seem to subside. On the other hand, bipolar disorder often occurs in intermittent episodes that are more or less determined by mood levels.

- **Triggered mood instability.** Individuals who have ADHD tend to be passionate, and have strong and emotional reactions to events happening around them. Whatever triggers the mood shifts with ADHD is different from what triggers the mood shifts in bipolar disorder. Happy circumstances in the lives of ADHD individuals tend to result in equally happy and elated states of mood. Likewise, unhappy circumstances resulting from rejection and criticism also result in a low mood.

Managing ADHD With Bipolar Disorder

At some point in our lives, we all are forced to cope with anger, anxiety, and impatience. Nevertheless, ADHD that is comorbid with bipolar disorder tends to magnify these emotions. In extreme cases, ever-changing moods can greatly interfere with careers, social interactions, and relationships. To cope with ADHD and bipolar, one should schedule appropriate times to vent, besides learning to take control of hyper-focus. Also, exercising more often will help removes negative energy.

Psychotherapy is often used alongside medical intervention to manage ADHD and bipolar disorder among kids and adults. You have to keep in mind the fact that even though medication alleviates some of the symptoms of ADHD and bipolar, individuals ought to make a deliberate effort to sign up for both individual therapy and psycho-education sessions. Psychotherapy classes typically entail teaching patients how to embrace their condition without feeling bitter about the impact that it might have had on their lives.

ADHD patients who are also finding it hard to complete tasks should also look to break them down into smaller portions. The completion of individual mini-tasks will give them a sense of accomplishment. What's more, it is advisable that adult ADHD individuals learn as much as they can about the disorder, since it will put them in a good position to face it.

Generally, a behavioral disorder affects job performance in various ways. If you cannot sit still during meetings, or if you have difficulties staying focused and organized, it will be hard for you to stay in one job for a substantial amount of time. Typically, individuals battling with ADHD and bipolar may have trouble with working memory, attention, verbal fluency, and mental processing. These qualities are generally referred to as executive-function abilities, and they come in handy at the workplace. Within the work environment, it is easy for you to get depressed or have low self-esteem if you have difficulties completing your tasks within schedules or beating simple deadlines. This may make your situation even worse.

The success of psychotherapy sessions for ADHD adults who also have bipolar starts with them remembering minor routines and keeping to the appointment time with the therapist. This is a step in the right direction, and will help them learn how to keep subsequent appointments with the therapist, and any other people that they are to meet in the future. Therapy for ADHD adults is done to help them know how best they can manage their condition. It similarly helps them learn how to change whatever long-standing poor self-image they might have. They do so by examining their experiences with the disorder in years gone by, and how to avoid the not-so-good ones.

Conclusion

ADHD is one of the most misunderstood behavioral disorders. Lots of myths and misconceptions exist pertaining to the disorder. In addition, it remains largely undetected in many people owing to the fact that its symptoms overlap with those of other mental disorders. There are also many myths and misconceptions about ADHD, something that has created confusion as what the condition really is, what causes it, and how it can be treated. Since ADHD affects many people, there is a need to raise awareness about it so that some of the misconceptions can be addressed.

Lastly, if you enjoyed this book I ask that you please take the time to review it on Audible.com. Your honest feedback would be greatly appreciated.

Thank you.

Now, I would like to share with you a free sneak peek to another one of my books that I think you will really enjoy. The book is called "Cognitive Behavioral Therapy (CBT): A Practical Guide to Free Yourself" Published by Lawrence M. Satterfield and Jason Wallace.

It's A Practical Guide to Learn the Most Effective CBT and DBT Techniques to Overcome Anxiety, Depression and Insomnia. You will also learn Exercises that will help you to Retrain your Brain and become more self-aware.

Enjoy!

The Mind with Cognitive Behavioral Therapy

will dig deeper into the practices of CBT and how you can benefit from them.

Firstly, it's important to understand how your brain responds to cognitive behavioral therapy. There have been some amazing studies on the matter. Not only does CBT affect your mind and the way you think, but it can also even affect how your brain operates as a biological function.

A group of researchers from universities in Sweden such as Linköping University decided to get together and study cognitive behavioral therapy. They did this because we have long known that the brain is incredibly adaptable. Some studies have even shown that activities such as video games and juggling can affect the volume of your brain.

To study how CBT affects the brain, the researchers conducted a study on a group of people by having them participate in cognitive behavioral therapy through the internet. One of the most common mental illnesses was the focus of this study. This illness is social anxiety disorder and affects an estimated fifteen million people within America.

Magnetic resonance imaging, commonly referred to as MRI, was conducted on all the participants both at the beginning and end of their CBT treatment. This study is amazing because not only do we have studies proving the mental effects of CBT, but this one is even looking at the biological effects.

In the initial brain scans, it was found that people with social anxiety disorder have an altered brain volume and the activity in a portion of their brain is increased. This portion of the brain is the amygdala, which is used primarily to make decisions, process memories, and emotional responses. It's easy to imagine how these changes could affect our mental state.

It may seem as if this biological function is out of our control, but this study proves otherwise. In fact, the study found that when the participants with social anxiety disorder completed nine weeks of CBT through the internet, their brains improved. These people experienced a reduction in brain volume and a decrease in the activity of the amygdala. The patients whose anxiety improved the most also experienced the greatest decrease in brain volume and amygdala activity.

This study proves the power of cognitive behavioral therapy. It isn't simply a false sense of positive thinking that some people may assume. Rather, it creates a real change in how you perceive the world, your reactions, your mood, and yes, even your brain.

What about people like Mary who suffers from debilitating depression? I have good news. Cognitive behavioral therapy has had great success on people living with depression. The results are amazing. CBT has been shown to be twice as effective as antidepressants in preventing depressive relapses.

The study which proved this was hoping to find the effects of both antidepressants and CBT on depressed people. While the researchers hypothesized that both treatments would treat depression similarly, they were surprised by the results.

Throughout treatment with some participants on antidepressants and others practicing cognitive behavioral therapy, the researchers would scan their brains with an MRI.

They were soon surprised to find that antidepressants and CBT impact completely different areas of the brain for people with depression. Antidepressants would reduce the activity in the emotional center of the brain known as the limbic system. Surprisingly, CBT helped to calm the area of the brain which is responsible for our reasoning, the cortex.

This means that while antidepressants reduce our emotions, CBT can actively help us to process them in a more proactive and healthy manner. This explains why CBT is much more effective in the long run and less likely to result in a depressive relapse down the road.

Post-traumatic stress disorder, often simply referred to as PTSD is a common condition which people suffer from after undergoing a traumatic event. Most people only consider veterans who went to war having PTSD. However, there are many other people who live every day with this condition. For instance, people who have undergone painful surgeries, those who have been in accidents, people who have lost someone close to them, and sexual assault victims. The symptoms of PTSD vary from person to person, but a few of the symptoms include:

- Flashbacks reliving a traumatic experience.
- Nightmares.
- Avoiding events, places, or objects that remind a person of the traumatic experience.
- Feeling tense, on edge, and easily startled.
- Experiencing angry outbursts.
- Having difficulty sleeping.
- Difficulty remembering or recalling the traumatic event.

- Guilt, blame, or other negative thoughts towards yourself.
- Loss of interest in your daily life and enjoyable activities.

There is much more, but these are some of the most common symptoms of PTSD. If you suspect you may have PTSD, please talk with a psychologist or psychiatrist and they can walk you through it. It is always recommended to get help from a trained professional who can personalize your care and treatment plan. However, this book can help alongside your doctor during your journey towards healing.

One study showing the effects of cognitive behavioral therapy was conducted with the participation of one-hundred children who were suffering from PTSD after being sexually assaulted. They had the children go into therapy, some with their mothers present and others with solely the therapist. Their condition was checked at regular intervals to see how the children were healing from the trauma.

The children completed tests both before, during, and after the treatment periods. After the original cognitive behavioral therapy, the children's tests scores improved significantly. These continued to improve over the following two years. This suggests that CBT is a successful treatment option for long-term improvement and care.

But in order to receive these benefits, it is important to understand in-depth how to utilize cognitive behavioral therapy. This therapy is a powerful tool and if you understand its basis and how to follow it through, you can experience amazing benefits.

While cognitive behavioral therapy involves some positive thinking, there is more to it than that. In fact, if you tell a person who is depressed, anxious, stressed, or suffering from trauma simply "just think positively," it will only cause them further stress. This is because positive thoughts alone are not enough to cause lasting change. When a person tries this and it doesn't work, they are likely to feel frustrated. This down-spiral further increases negative thoughts. Instead, it is important to practice using your mind as a tool over your mood. This will help you to consider all the information you have access to from various angles. If you are able to consider a situation (whether negative or positive) from all sides, then you can find a new understanding and solutions to your problems.

A good example of this is Lydia. If she simply told herself "I won't have anxiety when I see the neighbor's dog. I'm perfectly fine," she would be unrealistic and wouldn't be prepared for the anxiety she is likely to face once she sees the dog. Once she begins to feel anxiety upon seeing the dog, Lydia may end up feeling like a failure. Even a small amount of anxiety will make her feel as if there is no point to positive thinking.

Instead, Lydia will do better if she studies the situation from all sides and then decides on a solution for how to react if she becomes anxious. She can then think positively trusting in herself and her plan to help get her through coming across dogs. This is more successful because if we only allow false positive thoughts, then we will be unprepared for difficult situations.

Identifying your thoughts and then analyzing, testing, considering alternatives, and using your mind over your mood are important aspects of CBT. Although it is equally important to make behavioral changes along with these, it is important to keep in mind that cognitive behavioral therapy is consists of many components. Just like the inner pieces of a clock, CBT is only successful when all of the parts are working together.

Work on identifying your thoughts and analyzing them, thinking more positively, coming up with plans to reduce anxiety, and more. But also makes changes in your life. These changes will vary from person to person.

Rather than avoiding all dogs, Lydia could try acclimating to friendly small dogs until she feels comfortable. This will help her overcome her fear overtime and learn how to better manage her anxiety.

Mary needs to make a point of communicating with friends and spending time doing enjoyable activities. Her depression may make her feel like doing nothing but lying in bed and staring at the ceiling. But in order to improve the depression, she needs to get back out into life.

With Matt's alcoholism, he shouldn't keep alcohol around the house or go to bars. Instead, he needs to make a goal of becoming sober and attend regular meetings for alcoholics.

Likewise, if someone is being abused, they shouldn't simply "think happy thoughts" and become more submissive to their oppressor. Instead, their focus should be on finding a safe way to escape the abusive situation.

Now that you understand that this process is not solely about a false and short lasting positive thinking, it is time to address our negative thought processes. These thoughts control our actions in many ways. Maybe you were too scared to follow the career of your dreams because you might fail. Perhaps you become so overwhelmed that you procrastinate constantly. Or maybe you begin binge eating because you ate a single cookie and feel like a failure so what even is the point? All of these negative thoughts and more are damaging. Over time, they not only prevent us from attaining our goals and the life we desire, but they also will increasingly affect our mental health.

This is because of our negative thoughts and circumstances will accumulate. This shows in Lydia's story, where her trauma of dogs didn't surface until after she had been through a stressful divorce, move, and promotion. After all of the negative thoughts and emotions of the past year accumulated, she was unable to handle the anxiety and it manifested by bringing back her childhood trauma.

These thoughts can also combine in ways that make us think more negatively of ourselves such as in Matt's case, or as if there is no point in doing anything, like with Mary.

It is important to recognize all of your negative thoughts and learn to analyze and test them and then overcome them. But to do that, first, you need to know how to recognize them. There are ten main types of negative thoughts. Many people will experience most, if not all of these from time to time. But people often fall into centering on one or two types of negative thoughts.

These include:

1. Focusing on the Negative: *"Everything always goes wrong, life is just one disappointment after another."*
2. Negative Labeling of Yourself: *"I'm a terrible person and a failure. If people knew who I really was, they would leave me."*
3. Perfectionism: *"I have to do everything perfectly, otherwise I am a failure. I can't let anyone see anything of mine unless it's perfect."*
4. Constant Approval Needed: *"I have to make everyone like me. That's the only way I can be happy."*

5. Worst Case Scenario: *"Everything is going to be a disaster. It can't go well. I'm doomed."*

6. Ignoring the Present: *"I'll take care of myself later. For now, I have a list of things to accomplish."*

7. Other People Should Do What I Think: *"My friend shouldn't be posting so many photos of her boyfriend on social media. My adult daughter shouldn't be pursuing that career. That stranger shouldn't be wearing that, it's unflattering."*

8. Mind Reader: *"Other people must hate me, otherwise they wouldn't behave that way."*

9. Living in the Past: *"I'm miserable. I'm going to lay here and think about what happened to make me feel this way."*

10. Glass Half Empty: *"I don't trust people who are happy. If anything good ever happens in my life, then it is all going to be destroyed."*

The thoughts will vary from person to person depending on their situation. But most people will fit into at least one or two of these categories. After we figure out how we think, we can begin to counteract it. To do this, we start by finding the deceptions within those thought patterns.

Keep a little notebook with you or simply use a smartphone and keep track of your negative thoughts. You want a list that resembles sections titled:

- Situation
- Mood
- Automatic Thoughts or Images
- Evidence that Supports my Thoughts

- Evidence that Disproves my Thoughts
- Alternative Healthy Thoughts
- New Mood

When creating this list, you should use the four W's to help you. This means always fill out who, what, when, and where. You want to be specific, because if you simply state that it was happening "all day," then you are unable to target the cause behind the feelings. But if you know that you felt this way at 8:30 am when you were on your way to work, this narrows things down greatly.

Under the mood column, write any and all of the moods you were feeling at the time. You may have been feeling overwhelmed, depressed, anxious, sad, hurt, nervous, angry, or other emotions. When listing these, it is beneficial to rate them on a score of zero to one-hundred. These allow people who experience panic or anxiety attacks to log the severity.

Under the automatic thoughts or images, write any of the thoughts that were going through your head at the time. Taking the example from a moment ago, imagine that the thoughts running through your mind on the way to work that triggered this were *"I'm going to be late," "They'll fire me and then I won't have a job,"* and *"I'm worthless"*. If these thoughts were running through your head, you would write them down in this column and then analyze them in the following columns.

Next, tie together the columns for automatic thoughts and mood together on a rating of zero to one-hundred. For each thought, rate how it made you feel. Did the thought of being late makes you twenty percent anxious? The thought of being fired and without a job eighty percent scared? The thought of being worthless ninety percent depressed? By ranking the emotions tied to each of these thoughts, you can learn to better recognize damaging thoughts and proceed to overcome them.

The following step is one of the most important in this method and that is analyzing the evidence on whether or not your feelings are true or false. This can help us learn to identify what is a fact rather than our interpretation of a situation. There are many questions you can ask yourself to analyze these thoughts, but in the example we have been exploring, you might ask "Do I know I won't make it to work on time," "Are they likely to fire someone for being late once," "am I blaming myself for something out of my control," "When I'm not feeling this way, what do I think of this situation," "Are there any positives about myself that I am ignoring", and "If my best friend knew how I was feeling, what would they say?"

After analyzing the thought, you can fill in the alternative healthy thought section. Here, if you found that your thoughts weren't true, then you could fill in a more accurate thought. This might be "I haven't been late this year and my boss loves me, they are unlikely to fire me. I know I'm not worthless, every person has value and I have learned to be kind and compassionate. I am a valuable person"

If your thoughts were partially true, take the new information to write a more balanced view. For instance "my boss won't be happy, but I doubt I will be without a job. I may have slept through my alarm this morning, but that doesn't negate my intrinsic worth as a human being. I can take steps to wake up on time in the future."

After you analyze your thoughts and create new healthier and more balanced thoughts, you can rate how the new thoughts make you feel on a level of zero to one-hundred like you did with the original thought.

While this forum will change moment by moment for any given person, depending on the situations they are going through, let's look at what it might look like if Mary and Matt filled out this forum.

Mary:

- **Situation:**
  Didn't answer the phone when a friend called at noon.

- **Mood:**
  Depressed ninety percent, anxious thirty percent, worthlessness fifty percent.

- **Automatic Thoughts or Images:**
  "I can't be close to people. If I am, they'll die and I'll lose them," "I'm bad luck to have around," "Why am I even alive?"

- **Evidence that Supports my Thoughts:**
  My loved ones keep dying.

- **Evidence that Disproves my Thoughts:**
  Death is a part of life.
  My friends and pets were ill.
  I cared for them as best as I could do while they were alive.
  Their deaths were out of my hands.
  People aren't bad or good luck.
  Everyone is alive for a purpose.
  My friends care about me and want me around.

- **Alternative Healthy Thoughts:**
  "I'm sad that they died, but it wasn't my fault and I can't blame myself. My friends care about me and if I wasn't around, they would be sad."

- **New Mood:**
  Depressed forty percent, sad twenty percent, hopeful twenty percent.

As you can see, Mary may not feel all better, but she is working through her emotions. Her thoughts and mood are more stable now and she is reminded of why she is alive.

Now, let's look at Matt:

- **Situation:**
  His ex-girlfriend came by for a box of her stuff at 6 pm.

- **Mood:**
  Angry eighty percent, sad fifty percent.

- **Automatic Thoughts or Images:**
  "Why did she have to come by tonight when I was already having a bad day? She should have known it was too soon to see each other, now I miss her even more. This is her fault. If she had only forgiven me. I want a drink."

- **Evidence that Supports my Thoughts:**
  I apologized, she could have forgiven me.

- **Evidence that Disproves my Thoughts:**
  She needed her stuff and had a right to come get it. Even after the breakup, she was being kind and asked how I was doing.
  The breakup isn't her fault. She stuck with me for two years despite my drinking and anger.
  She doesn't have to forgive me and even if she has, that doesn't mean she is required to stay with me.

- **Alternative Healthy Thoughts:**
  "I'm sad that we broke up, but I hope she lives a happy

life. Now that I am single, I can focus on bettering my own life, becoming sober, and controlling my temper. This is better for both of us in the long-run. A drink won't help me and I want to stay sober."

- **New Mood:**
  Sad fifteen percent, encouraged twenty percent, motivated fifty percent.

While Matt began the process as angry, as he worked through his feelings, whether they were true or false and developed a healthier alternative thought, he was able to work through his anger. This helped him to accept the breakup at the moment and encouraged him to stay sober. He may struggle with his anger and the breakup from time to time in the future, but if he continues to get through it in this healthy manner, then he can improve his life, learn to control his anger, and resist alcohol. Over time, the breakup will begin to hurt less.

It is important to retain awareness of your own mental state. To do this, try to fill out this forum regularly, especially whenever you notice your mood is low or your thoughts are destructive. But sometimes it can be hard to start because we are greatly lacking an awareness of our thoughts. This can be especially true when we have been living with a condition such as depression or anxiety for a long time. We become so accustomed to it that it turns into background noise. We need to learn to listen into this background noise so that we can tune it into a beautiful melody rather than a high-pitched static. Asking different questions based on our moods can help.

Generalized questions are a good place to start because you can ask them of yourself, no matter what your mood is. You may find it difficult to place a finger on exactly what you had been thinking of prior to a mood shift, but with some time, you will become an expert at realizing and recalling what is impacting your mood. After practice, many people will be able to place their finger on what upset them simply by answering these two questions:

- What was the last thing going through my mind before I noticed my mood shift?
- What memories or images was I experiencing?

The second question is regarding images and memories because many people find that their strongest mood shifts aren't a response to a specific thought. Rather, it was a response to a memory or image they thought of. For instance, for a split second, someone could remember a still image of a loved one in the hospital. If you have a lot going on in your life, it is easy to get distracted and not remember what triggered it, but the negative emotions remain. This is why it's important to learn to target and analyze what is affecting you.

After answering the generalized questions, you can answer some more specific mood-related questions.

When people are anxious, they often consider worst-case scenarios of what could happen in the near or distant future. We overestimate what could go wrong while simultaneously underestimating ourselves. When you find yourself anxious, scared, or nervous, then ask yourself *"what am I afraid might happen?"* and *"what is the worst that could happen?"*

If you find yourself depressed, it is easy to be self-critical or even hate yourself completely. In this case, it's easy to not just be critical about ourselves, but life in general as well. Therefore, if you are feeling depressed, sad, discouraged, or disappointed, I want you to ask yourself three questions. *"What does this mean about me?"*, *"What does this mean about my future?"*, and *"What does this mean about life?"*

People often feel guilt or shame in conjunction with their actions even if they didn't do anything wrong. For instance, people can have survivor's guilt if someone close to them died yet they survived. There was nothing wrong with them surviving and they couldn't have saved the other person, yet they feel guilty. Though these feelings can, of course, have validity as well. If you got into a fight with your sibling, you could feel guilty for something you said. If you find yourself feeling this way, ask yourself *"Did I hurt someone, break a law/rule, not have done something I should have, or otherwise gone against my moral code?"*, *"What does this mean about how others feel about me?"*, *"What do I think or believe about myself?"*, and *"What would other people think if they knew?"*

We can often feel angry, irritated, or resentful if we have felt as if someone has harmed us in some way. Even if the person wasn't unjust or mistreating us, we can often feel antsy from anger. It is important to distinguish whether or not this anger is justified. There is righteous anger. For instance, we can be angry when we learn of a child being abused. Non-righteous anger would be us getting angry that the cheeseburger that we ordered had pickles when we asked for no pickles. Sure, the person who made the cheeseburger made a mistake, but it is not something to get upset about if they are willing to fix it for us. If you are having anger related feelings, ask yourself *"What does this mean about other people?"* and *"What does this mean about how other people feel about me?"*

By asking yourself these questions, you will learn to recognize your emotions and the thoughts, memories, and images that trigger them. While what other people do and say can impact our emotions, remember that it is ultimately how we respond to those people that impact our long-term emotional state.

Occasionally, you may want to try looking over some of the other questions that aren't in your emotional category. For instance, if you are feeling anxious, you still may benefit by asking yourself the depression questions. Over time, you may even develop some of your own questions which you find is helping you to identify why you are feeling or reacting in specific ways.

Thank you, this preview is now over.

I hope you enjoyed this preview of my book Cognitive Behavioral Therapy (CBT).

Please make sure to check out the full book on Amazon.com

Thank you.

www.ingramcontent.com/pod-product-compliance
Lightning Source LLC
Chambersburg PA
CBHW031148020426
42333CB00013B/557